# Effective Media Communication during Public Health Emergencies

## A WHO HANDBOOK

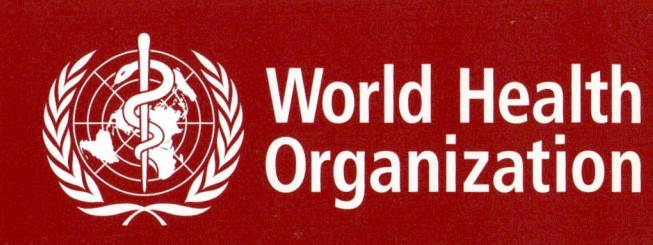

Geneva, 2007

WHO Library Cataloguing-in-Publication Data

Hyer, Randall N.
    Effective media communication during public health emergencies : a WHO handbook / Randall N. Hyer, Vincent T. Covello.

    1.Disease outbreaks 2.Communications media 3.Mass media 4.Public relations 5.Manuals 6.Guidelines I.Covello, Vincent T. II.World Health Organization.

    ISBN 92 4 154703 0             (NLM classification: WA 110)
    ISBN 978 92 4 154703 1

## © World Health Organization 2007

All rights reserved. Publications of the World Health Organization can be obtained from WHO Press, World Health Organization, 20 Avenue Appia, 1211 Geneva 27, Switzerland (tel: +41 22 791 3264; fax: +41 22 791 4857; e-mail: bookorders@who.int). Requests for permission to reproduce or translate WHO publications – whether for sale or for noncommercial distribution – should be addressed to WHO Press, at the above address (fax: +41 22 791 4806; e-mail: permissions@who.int).

The designations employed and the presentation of the material in this publication do not imply the expression of any opinion whatsoever on the part of the World Health Organization concerning the legal status of any country, territory, city or area or of its authorities, or concerning the delimitation of its frontiers or boundaries. Dotted lines on maps represent approximate border lines for which there may not yet be full agreement.

The mention of specific companies or of certain manufacturers' products does not imply that they are endorsed or recommended by the World Health Organization in preference to others of a similar nature that are not mentioned. Errors and omissions excepted, the names of proprietary products are distinguished by initial capital letters.

All reasonable precautions have been taken by the World Health Organization to verify the information contained in this publication. However, the published material is being distributed without warranty of any kind, either expressed or implied. The responsibility for the interpretation and use of the material lies with the reader. In no event shall the World Health Organization be liable for damages arising from its use.

The named authors alone are responsible for the views expressed in this publication.

Printed in France

**Randall N Hyer** MD, PhD, MPH

Medical Officer, Alert and Response Operations
Department of Communicable Disease Surveillance and Response
World Health Organization
Geneva, Switzerland

**Vincent T Covello** PhD

Director
Center for Risk Communication
New York City
United States of America

## Acknowledgements

This handbook has been drawn from a wide variety of sources, including articles by the above authors, and documents and articles produced by WHO Member States, regional offices and country offices. Special thanks are also given to the following individuals:

| | | |
|---|---|---|
| Tomas Allen | DA Henderson | Mike Ryan |
| Robert Alvey | Michael Hopmeier | Cristina Salvi |
| Ann Andersen | Richard Hyde | Ron Sconyers |
| Bret Atkins | Margaret Joseph | Monica Shoch-Spalla |
| Maurizio Babeschi | Mary Kay Kindhauser | Mary Ann Simmons |
| Kazem Behbehani | Jennifer Leaning | Iain Simpson |
| Samantha Bloem | Clem Levin | Gloria Tam |
| Brian Butler | Expedito de Albuquerque Luna | Kiyosu Taniguchi |
| Mike Cameron | Craig Manning | Dick Thompson |
| Elaine Chatigny | Malin Modh | Timothy Tinker |
| John Clements | Karen Morrione | Belinda Towns |
| Ottorino Cosivi | Sandra Mullin | Robert Ulmer |
| Peggy Creese | David Nabarro | TE van Deventer |
| David Degagne | Rafael Obregon | Marsha Vanderford |
| Ellen Egan | Sam Okware | Mark Vanommeren |
| Gaya Gamhewage | Sam Page | Dave Wade |
| Donna Garland | Richard Peters | Myron Weinberg |
| Mohamed Mehdi Gouya | Lisa Pogoff | Joseph Wojtecki |
| John Grabenstein | Maura Ricketts | Sally Young |
| Gregory Hartl | David Ropeik | Maria Zampaglione |
| Mike Heideman | Dan Rutz | |

Acknowledgement is also given to Anthony L Waddell for his expert editing of the text, as well as to Threefold Design Ltd for the design layout.

# PREFACE

In recent years public health agencies have considerably improved their ability to rapidly detect and respond to public health emergencies. At the same time, mechanisms for global cooperation and resource pooling have been greatly strengthened. Despite these advances, effectively communicating the threats posed by such emergencies and the actions needed during them remains a significant challenge. Such communication needs to be carefully planned and implemented as well as properly integrated with emergency management activities and operations. To communicate effectively through the media during a public health emergency, response managers must plan their communication strategies, integrate communicators into the most senior levels, provide transparent messages, and listen to the public's concerns.

Emergency events therefore present a unique challenge to the internal media-relations capabilities of health agencies. Although such events are hard to predict, media communication strategies for them can be planned in advance. Prior approval of communication strategies helps to minimize secondary damage (such as adverse economic or political effects) and leads to greater trust. Such advance planning also greatly increases the likelihood that the resulting news media coverage will further public health interests and contribute positively to emergency response efforts. Well-constructed and properly delivered media messages can inform and calm a worried public, reduce misinformation, and focus attention on what is most important.

Effective media communication is clearly a key responsibility of public health professionals. It is all too easy to be caught unprepared, especially for short-notice or demanding media interviews, and preparation is vital. Communicate badly and one may be perceived as incompetent, uncaring or dishonest. Communicate well and one can reach more people with a clear and credible public health message.

This handbook describes a seven-step process to assist public health officials and others to communicate effectively through the media during emergencies. At the core of this process is the belief that positive action must be taken to interactively facilitate effective media coverage of events and situations rather than simply responding to the resulting coverage. By implementing such a "proactive" and interactive approach, public health organizations and officials will be in a stronger position to ensure that their messages are accurately reported, highly visible and clearly heard. This will greatly increase the likelihood of successfully informing people, encouraging helpful behaviours by those affected or threatened, and significantly reducing the impact of events.

Although presented sequentially, all seven steps are in fact inter-dependent and form a continuous loop. In particular, the final step of evaluation is an ongoing and almost constant process aimed at improving communication activities at all steps based on feedback. Agencies and organizations should take every opportunity to obtain and apply feedback. Lessons should be learned and implemented to improve performance both immediately and in the long term.

The handbook is aimed at WHO office and field personnel who are unfamiliar with media interactions or who wish to sharpen their skills in this area. It is also intended to help public health officials in other organizations and networks to deal with the media communication aspects of emergencies. As an aid to easy recollection of the key issues in this area, a double-sided wall chart has been provided to accompany this handbook. The chart shows the seven-step approach and provides easily recalled key information and advice.

Although it covers many issues, this handbook is primarily intended to serve as a reference during planning sessions and as a reminder of key points. It can also be used as a training and preparation tool. Effectively communicating through the media is a learned skill that requires training and practice. Even in our diverse and culturally rich global community, there are universal and commonly accepted best practices for effective media communication. These best practices are supported by a robust scientific evidence base, which includes documented consequences of *not* using best practices. Global best practices and principles should always be tailored to local needs, and this handbook should be complemented with local and regional media training. It is recognized that many of the tasks described are ideals and may be difficult to put into practice. This will be especially true where the human and financial resources needed are not available.

The main focus of this handbook is on the news media as a means to reach people and on the interactions with journalists necessary to achieve this. Consequently, it offers only limited guidance on face-to-face exchanges or dialogues with the public during emergency events. Readers wishing to pursue this topic should consult texts dedicated to offering guidance on interactive exchanges with the public in emergency and non-emergency situations. In general, working with the media during an emergency must be recognized as only one aspect of a larger overall communication strategy. This handbook is not a description of how to develop and implement such a strategy. Nor does it describe how to develop and implement advocacy or social marketing campaigns, as these are largely the provinces of health educators or social mobilization specialists.

A separate WHO "field guide" has been produced that highlights the practical aspects of the seven-step approach described in full in this handbook. The field guide can act as a rapid primer document as it covers media communication activities that are crucially important during a public health emergency.

# TABLE OF CONTENTS

LIST OF FIGURES, TABLES, BOXES AND INFORMATION POINTS — vi

**INTRODUCTION** — viii

### STEP 1: Assess media needs, media constraints, and internal media-relations capabilities
- **1.1:** ASSESS THE NEEDS OF THE MEDIA — 1
- **1.2:** ASSESS THE CONSTRAINTS OF THE MEDIA — 5
- **1.3:** ASSESS INTERNAL MEDIA-RELATIONS CAPABILITIES — 8

### STEP 2: Develop goals, plans and strategies
- **2.1:** DEVELOP MEDIA COMMUNICATION GOALS AND OBJECTIVES — 11
- **2.2:** DEVELOP A WRITTEN MEDIA COMMUNICATION PLAN — 13
- **2.3:** DEVELOP A PARTNER AND STAKEHOLDER STRATEGY — 20

### STEP 3: Train communicators
- **3.1:** TRAIN THE MEDIA COMMUNICATION TEAM — 25
- **3.2:** TRAIN A PUBLIC INFORMATION OFFICER — 27
- **3.3:** TRAIN A DESIGNATED LEAD SPOKESPERSON — 28

### STEP 4: Prepare messages
- **4.1:** PREPARE LISTS OF STAKEHOLDERS AND THEIR CONCERNS — 35
- **4.2:** PREPARE CLEAR AND CONCISE MESSAGES — 39
- **4.3:** PREPARE TARGETED MESSAGES — 48

### STEP 5: Identify media outlets and media activities
- **5.1:** IDENTIFY AVAILABLE MEDIA OUTLETS — 51
- **5.2:** IDENTIFY THE MOST EFFECTIVE MEDIA OUTLETS — 54
- **5.3:** IDENTIFY MEDIA ACTIVITIES FOR THE FIRST 24–72 HOURS — 60

### STEP 6: Deliver messages
- **6.1:** DELIVER CLEAR AND TIMELY MESSAGES — 65
- **6.2:** DELIVER MESSAGES TO MAINTAIN VISIBILITY — 69
- **6.3:** DELIVER TARGETED MESSAGES — 73

### STEP 7: Evaluate messages and performance
- **7.1:** EVALUATE MESSAGE DELIVERY AND MEDIA COVERAGE — 77
- **7.2:** EVALUATE AND IMPROVE PERFORMANCE BASED ON FEEDBACK — 81
- **7.3:** EVALUATE PUBLIC RESPONSES TO MESSAGES — 85

## ANNEXES

**ANNEX 1.** REFLECTING CULTURAL DIVERSITY IN COMMUNICATION ACTIVITIES AND MATERIALS — 87

**ANNEX 2.** WHO OUTBREAK COMMUNICATION GUIDELINES — 90

**ANNEX 3.** PRINCIPLES AND TECHNIQUES OF EFFECTIVE MEDIA COMMUNICATION — 95

**ANNEX 4.** SAMPLE MEDIA COMMUNICATION PLAN CONTENTS — 100

**ANNEX 5.** SAMPLE LETTER OF ENDORSEMENT BY THE AGENCY DIRECTOR OF THE MEDIA COMMUNICATION PLAN — 101

**ANNEX 6.** QUESTIONS FREQUENTLY ASKED BY JOURNALISTS AND THE PUBLIC DURING DISEASE OUTBREAKS — 102

**ANNEX 7.** EFFECTIVELY COMMUNICATING RISK NUMBERS — 105

**ANNEX 8.** FACTORS IN RISK PERCEPTION — 110

**ANNEX 9.** HOW PEOPLE FORM RISK PERCEPTIONS AND MAKE RISK JUDGEMENTS — 112

**ANNEX 10.** HOW PEOPLE PROCESS RISK INFORMATION IN HIGH-STRESS SITUATIONS — 114

**ANNEX 11.** HOW PEOPLE FORM PERCEPTIONS OF TRUST — 115

## SELECTED READING

INTERNATIONAL PERSPECTIVES AND CULTURAL DIVERSITY — 116

HEALTH, RISK AND EMERGENCY COMMUNICATIONS — 118

MEDIA COMMUNICATION AND PUBLIC HEALTH — 122

# LIST OF FIGURES, TABLES, BOXES AND INFORMATION POINTS

## INTRODUCTION

| | |
|---|---:|
| **FIGURE ONE:** SEVEN STEPS TO EFFECTIVE MEDIA COMMUNICATION DURING PUBLIC HEALTH EMERGENCIES | xi |
| **INFORMATION POINT:** Cross-cultural sensitivity in message design | ix |

## STEP 1: ASSESS MEDIA NEEDS, MEDIA CONSTRAINTS, AND INTERNAL MEDIA-RELATIONS CAPABILITIES

| | |
|---|---:|
| **BOX 1.1:** 77 MOST FREQUENTLY ASKED QUESTIONS BY JOURNALISTS IN AN EMERGENCY | 2 |
| **BOX 1.2:** INTERNAL MEDIA-RELATIONS CAPABILITIES – AN ASSESSMENT TOOL | 8 |
| **INFORMATION POINT:** Questions to ask as part of assessing internal media-relations capabilities before, during and after an emergency | 10 |

## STEP 2: DEVELOP GOALS, PLANS AND STRATEGIES

| | |
|---|---:|
| **BOX 2.1:** PANIC AVOIDANCE AS A GOAL | 11 |
| **BOX 2.2:** EXAMPLE OF A MEDIA COMMUNICATION GOAL STATEMENT | 12 |
| **BOX 2.3:** BASIC INFORMATION TYPICALLY INCLUDED IN A MEDIA COMMUNICATION PLAN | 14 |
| **BOX 2.4:** ELEMENTS OF ORGANIZATIONAL CULTURE | 21 |
| **BOX 2.5:** ESTABLISHING WORKING RELATIONSHIPS WITH THE MEDIA BEFORE AN EMERGENCY OCCURS | 21 |
| **FIGURE TWO:** WORKSHEET FOR IDENTIFYING ORGANIZATIONS AND INDIVIDUALS TO BE CONTACTED DURING AN EMERGENCY | 15 |
| **INFORMATION POINT:** Considerations when developing relationships with partners | 22 |
| **INFORMATION POINT:** Common mistakes in working with partners | 22 |
| **INFORMATION POINT:** Working with partners | 23 |

## STEP 3: TRAIN COMMUNICATORS

| | |
|---|---:|
| **BOX 3.1:** MEDIA COMMUNICATION COMPETENCIES OF PUBLIC INFORMATION OFFICERS | 27 |
| **BOX 3.2:** PERSONAL AND PROFESSIONAL CHARACTERISTICS OF A DESIGNATED LEAD SPOKESPERSON | 28 |
| **BOX 3.3:** RECOMMENDED APPROACHES FOR LEAD AND OTHER SPOKESPERSONS WHEN DEALING WITH THE MEDIA DURING AN EMERGENCY | 29 |
| **BOX 3.4:** PITFALLS TO AVOID WHEN COMMUNICATING WITH THE MEDIA DURING AN EMERGENCY | 30 |
| **BOX 3.5:** NEGATIVELY PERCEIVED NON-VERBAL COMMUNICATION | 32 |
| **BOX 3.6:** POSITIVELY PERCEIVED NON-VERBAL COMMUNICATION | 33 |

## STEP 4: PREPARE MESSAGES

| | |
|---|---:|
| **BOX 4.1:** EXAMPLES OF STAKEHOLDERS DURING A MAJOR DISEASE OUTBREAK | 36 |
| **BOX 4.2:** POTENTIAL CONCERNS IN A PUBLIC HEALTH EMERGENCY | 37 |
| **BOX 4.3:** A FIVE-STEP MODEL FOR PREPARING MESSAGES FOR POTENTIAL MEDIA INTERVIEWS DURING AN EMERGENCY | 45 |
| **BOX 4.4:** RISK-PERCEPTION AND FEAR FACTORS | 47 |
| **FIGURE THREE:** MATRIX OF STAKEHOLDERS AND THEIR CONCERNS | 38 |
| **FIGURE FOUR:** MESSAGE MAP TEMPLATE | 40 |
| **FIGURE FIVE:** SAMPLE SMALLPOX MESSAGE MAP – WITH KEYWORDS IN ITALICS | 41 |
| **FIGURE SIX:** SAMPLE NEWS RELEASE TEMPLATE | 44 |
| **INFORMATION POINT:** Examples of technical terms used in public health that may not be understood by the public | 42 |
| **INFORMATION POINT:** Contents of a news release | 43 |
| **INFORMATION POINT:** Guidelines for preparing clear and concise messages during public health emergencies | 47 |
| **INFORMATION POINT:** Summary guidelines for simplifying interviews, presentations and messages | 49 |
| **INFORMATION POINT:** Communicating effectively to individuals experiencing extreme stress or anxiety | 50 |

## STEP 5: IDENTIFY MEDIA OUTLETS AND MEDIA ACTIVITIES

| | |
|---|---|
| **BOX 5.1:** ANTICIPATING AND PREPARING FOR AN EMERGENCY | 61 |
| **BOX 5.2:** ACTIVITY GUIDELINES FOR THE FIRST 24–72 HOURS AFTER NOTIFICATION AND VERIFICATION OF A PUBLIC HEALTH EMERGENCY | 62 |
| **FIGURE SEVEN:** IDENTIFYING AND PROFILING MEDIA OUTLETS | 53 |
| **FIGURE EIGHT:** WORKSHEET FOR TRACKING ENQUIRIES WITHIN THE FIRST 24–72 HOURS OF AN EMERGENCY | 63 |
| **INFORMATION POINT:** Causes of public health emergencies | 60 |

## STEP 6: DELIVER MESSAGES

| | |
|---|---|
| **BOX 6.1:** THE 33 MOST FREQUENTLY USED BRIDGING STATEMENTS | 68 |
| **BOX 6.2:** CORRECTING ERRORS IN MEDIA REPORTING | 72 |
| **BOX 6.3:** STRATEGIES FOR DELIVERING TARGETED MESSAGES | 73 |
| **BOX 6.4:** EXAMPLES OF TOPIC-RELATED QUESTIONS TO ASK A REPORTER BEFORE A MEDIA INTERVIEW | 74 |
| **BOX 6.5:** EXAMPLES OF PROCEDURAL QUESTIONS TO ASK A REPORTER BEFORE A MEDIA INTERVIEW | 75 |
| **INFORMATION POINT:** Contents of a media kit or packet | 71 |
| **INFORMATION POINT:** Holding a news conference | 72 |

## STEP 7: EVALUATE MESSAGES AND PERFORMANCE

| | |
|---|---|
| **BOX 7.1:** EVALUATING OPENNESS AND TRANSPARENCY OF COMMUNICATIONS | 77 |
| **BOX 7.2:** EVALUATING LISTENING | 78 |
| **BOX 7.3:** EVALUATING CLARITY | 78 |
| **BOX 7.4:** EVALUATION OF MEDIA COVERAGE | 79 |
| **BOX 7.5:** TYPES OF EVALUATION | 80 |
| **BOX 7.6:** EVALUATING SYSTEM PERFORMANCE – MEDIA COMMUNICATION PLANNING | 81 |
| **BOX 7.7:** EVALUATING SYSTEM PERFORMANCE – WORKING WITH THE MEDIA AND MEETING THE MEDIA'S FUNCTIONAL NEEDS | 82 |
| **BOX 7.8:** EVALUATING SYSTEM PERFORMANCE – COORDINATION ACTIVITIES | 83 |
| **BOX 7.9:** EVALUATING SYSTEM PERFORMANCE – MEDIA AND OUTREACH TASKS | 83 |
| **BOX 7.10:** EVALUATING SYSTEM PERFORMANCE – HOTLINES AND WEB SITES | 84 |
| **BOX 7.11:** EVALUATING OUTCOME MEASURES | 85 |
| **INFORMATION POINT:** Examples of process evaluation measures | 80 |
| **INFORMATION POINT:** Examples of outcome evaluation measures | 80 |

## ANNEX 1. REFLECTING CULTURAL DIVERSITY IN COMMUNICATION ACTIVITIES AND MATERIALS

| | |
|---|---|
| **BOX A:** GUIDELINES ON PLANNING AND IMPLEMENTING AN EFFECTIVE AND CULTURALLY SENSITIVE MEDIA PROGRAMME | 89 |

## ANNEX 7. EFFECTIVELY COMMUNICATING RISK NUMBERS

| | |
|---|---|
| **TABLE ONE:** Concentration comparisons | 108 |
| **TABLE TWO:** Various annual and lifetime risks | 109 |

## ANNEX 9. HOW PEOPLE FORM RISK PERCEPTIONS AND MAKE RISK JUDGEMENTS

| | |
|---|---|
| **FIGURE NINE:** FACTORS AFFECTING RISK PERCEPTION | 113 |

# INTRODUCTION

*We have had great success in the [last] five years in controlling outbreaks, but we have only recently come to understand that communications are as critical to outbreak control as laboratory analyses or epidemiology.*

Dr Jong-wook Lee, Director-General, WHO, 21 September 2004

Until the outbreak of an exotic communicable disease or other dramatic event, the elaborate infrastructures and mechanisms that protect public health on a daily basis often go unnoticed and attract little media[1] interest. In the midst of a public health emergency[2] the situation becomes very different as the demand for information rapidly escalates. Only recently has the true extent to which media communication[3] directly influences the course of events been recognized. Good communication can rally support, calm a nervous public, provide much-needed information, encourage cooperative behaviours and help save lives. Poor communication can fan emotions, disrupt economies and undermine confidence.

Recent outbreaks of severe acute respiratory syndrome (SARS) and avian influenza, releases of anthrax and sarin, and natural disasters such as the South-East Asian tsunami, underline the importance of communication during public health emergencies. Communication challenges are particularly pronounced when fear of a naturally occurring or deliberately released pathogen spreads faster and further than the resulting disease itself. In such situations, policy-makers, the news media and the public all expect timely and accurate information. It is vital that people feel that officials are communicating openly and honestly. The most important asset in any large-scale public health emergency is the public because ultimately they must take care of themselves. Through effective media communication, public health officials can engage the public and help them to make informed and better decisions.

Such effective media communication requires trust and understanding between public health officials and the media. The media depend on public health officials for timely and accurate information. Public health officials depend on the media to get their messages out before, during and after an emergency. They also use the media as a surveillance system. For these reasons, each side depends upon the other to be successful. The media should therefore be viewed both as a crucial means of conveying information and as a component of outbreak surveillance.

Effective media communication is in fact a crucial element in effective emergency management and should assume a central role from the start. It establishes public confidence in the ability of an organization or government to deal with an emergency, and to bring about a satisfactory conclusion. Effective media communication is also integral to the larger process of information exchange aimed at eliciting trust and promoting understanding of the relevant issues or actions. Within the limits of available knowledge, good media communication aids such efforts by:

- building, maintaining or restoring trust;
- improving knowledge and understanding;
- guiding and encouraging appropriate attitudes, decisions, actions and behaviours; and
- encouraging collaboration and cooperation.

Numerous government reports[4] have highlighted the importance of communication in enabling people to make informed choices and to participate in deciding how risks should be managed. This can be achieved by explaining mandatory regulations, informing and advising people of the risks they themselves can control, or dissuading people from engaging in risky behaviour. Effective media communication provides the public with timely, accurate, clear, objective, consistent and complete risk information and is the starting point for creating an informed population that is:

- involved, interested, reasonable, thoughtful, solution-oriented, cooperative and collaborative;
- appropriately concerned about the risk; and
- more likely to take appropriate action.

While effective media communication always aims to strengthen trust, its specific objectives can vary. The intention in some situations may be to proactively raise awareness of actual or potential risk, or to inform people prior to an emergency so they are better prepared to respond. In other cases, it may be a more reactive response to an existing situation. Other purposes include informing individuals and disseminating information on how to mitigate the effects of an emergency. In yet other cases, the purpose may be to build consensus and engage people in a public dialogue.

This handbook is organized around the seven-step process for guiding public health communicators in planning and implementing effective media communication shown in **FIGURE ONE**. Its primary focus is on relations with the news media (both print and broadcast) during a public health emergency – "media communication" can be taken to mean "news media communication". Many cultures, however, rely on folk and traditional[5] means of mass communication which typically originate from the beliefs, culture and customs of a specific population. As such, the handbook can be supplemented with materials, practices and guidance for specific localities and target populations. A guiding principle of effective media communication in a global context is that all communication activities and materials (including those prepared for the media) should reflect the diverse nature of societies in a fair, representative and inclusive manner.

---

**INFORMATION POINT: Cross-cultural sensitivity in message design**

Given the wide diversity of cultures, media communication should be sensitive to:
- words, images and situations that suggest cultural or ethnic stereotypes;
- negative implications of symbolism and usage that could offend people or reinforce bias;
- language with questionable racial or ethnic connotations;
- different cultural meanings assigned to:
  - symbols
  - signs
  - words;
- different cultural standards for:
  - attentiveness during conversation
  - distance between speakers during a conversation
  - what is considered humorous
  - what topics are considered inappropriate or taboo
  - taking turns during conversations
  - loudness, speed of delivery, length of delivery, silence, attentiveness and time to respond to another's point
  - entering into and exiting from conversations; and
- different meanings of colours and imagery.

**These considerations should be adapted to meet local needs**

1 **Media** – *the means of mass communication, especially television, radio, and newspapers collectively.* All text in italics taken from the *Compact Oxford English Dictionary of Current English*, Second Edition. Ed. C Soanes. Oxford University Press, Oxford, UK, 2003.
2 **Emergency** – *a serious, unexpected, and potentially dangerous situation requiring immediate action.*
3 **Communication** – *a means of sending or receiving information.* Also – the process by which information is exchanged between groups or individuals through mutually understood systems of language, symbols, signs, or behaviours.
4 Health and Safety Executive (1998). *Risk communication: a guide to regulatory practice.* Inter-Departmental Group on Risk Assessment, Health and Safety Executive, London.
National Research Council/National Academy of Sciences (1989). *Improving risk communication. Committee on Risk Perception and Risk Communication.* Washington, DC: National Academy Press.
Pan American Health Organization (1994). *Communicating with the public in times of disaster: guidelines for disaster managers on preparing and disseminating effective health messages.* Washington, DC.
Royal Society (1992). *Risk: analysis, perception, management.* Royal Society, London.
Swedish Emergency Management Agency (2003). *Crisis Communication Handbook.* Swedish Emergency Management Agency, Stockholm.
WHO (2004). *WHO Outbreak Communication Guidelines.* Geneva, World Health Organization.
5 **Folk and traditional media** – the means of mass communication *originating from the beliefs, culture, and customs* of a specific locality or population. Folk and traditional media include diverse and varied audio and visual forms such as storytelling, puppetry, songs, dancing, poetry recitals, sermons or the creative use of traditional arts and crafts.

## FIGURE ONE: SEVEN STEPS TO EFFECTIVE MEDIA COMMUNICATION DURING PUBLIC HEALTH EMERGENCIES

**STEP 1: Assess media needs, media constraints, and internal media-relations capabilities**
- **1.1:** *Assess* the needs of the media
- **1.2:** *Assess* the constraints of the media
- **1.3:** *Assess* internal media-relations capabilities

**STEP 2: Develop goals, plans and strategies**
- **2.1:** *Develop* media communication goals and objectives
- **2.2:** *Develop* a written media communication plan
- **2.3:** *Develop* a partner and stakeholder strategy

**STEP 3: Train communicators**
- **3.1:** *Train* the media communication team
- **3.2:** *Train* a public information officer
- **3.3:** *Train* a designated lead spokesperson

**STEP 4: Prepare messages**
- **4.1:** *Prepare* lists of stakeholders and their concerns
- **4.2:** *Prepare* clear and concise messages
- **4.3:** *Prepare* targeted messages

**STEP 5: Identify media outlets and media activities**
- **5.1:** *Identify* available media outlets
- **5.2:** *Identify* the most effective media outlets
- **5.3:** *Identify* media activities for the first 24–72 hours

**STEP 6: Deliver messages**
- **6.1:** *Deliver* clear and timely messages
- **6.2:** *Deliver* messages to maintain visibility
- **6.3:** *Deliver* targeted messages

**STEP 7: Evaluate messages and performance**
- **7.1:** *Evaluate* message delivery and media coverage
- **7.2:** *Evaluate* and improve performance based on feedback
- **7.3:** *Evaluate* public responses to messages

# STEP 1
## Assess media needs, media constraints, and internal media-relations capabilities

**1.1:** *Assess* the needs of the media
**1.2:** *Assess* the constraints of the media
**1.3:** *Assess* internal media-relations capabilities

# STEP 1
## Assess media needs, media constraints, and internal media-relations capabilities

**1.1:** *Assess* the needs of the media
**1.2:** *Assess* the constraints of the media
**1.3:** *Assess* internal media-relations capabilities

# 1.1: ASSESS THE NEEDS OF THE MEDIA

One must appreciate and meet the needs of the news media in order to advance one's agenda. News media include newspapers, magazines, television, radio and the internet. Understanding what the news media want from a story and what they are likely to ask helps to define what will best meet their needs (**BOX 1.1**). The news media can be valuable allies during an emergency.

## I. What do the news media typically do?

- gather and spread information;
- fulfil their commercial obligations (for example to make money for their owners or shareholders);
- compete with one another for news and ratings;
- act as a public "watchdog";
- search out interesting, newsworthy or sensational stories;
- inform and educate;
- interpret information;
- set public agendas or reflect what is already on the public agenda;
- attract listeners/viewers;
- reach large numbers of people; and
- express viewpoints.

## II. How can the news media help during an emergency?

- inform and educate;
- get the story out quickly;
- reach major target audiences;
- rally support;
- function as a public watchdog (for example by calling into question actions or recommendations);
- help prevent undue fear and anxiety;
- provide accurate and needed information;
- correct erroneous information;
- encourage appropriate behaviours; and
- calm a nervous public.

## III. What are news editors and producers typically looking for in a story?

- stories that increase ratings and profits by attracting large numbers of readers, viewers or listeners;
- stories that reflect the agendas or serve the interests of the editors, owners or publishers of media organizations;
- stories that help people understand issues so they can make informed choices;
- stories that serve the public interest; and
- stories that advance the personal career of the reporters.

STEP 1: Assess media needs, media constraints, and internal media-relations capabilities

### BOX 1.1: 77 MOST FREQUENTLY ASKED QUESTIONS BY JOURNALISTS IN AN EMERGENCY

1. What is your name and title?
2. How do you spell and pronounce your name?
3. What are your job responsibilities?
4. Can you tell us what happened? Were you there? How do you know what you are telling us?
5. When did it happen?
6. Where did it happen?
7. Who was harmed?
8. How many people were harmed?
9. Are those that were harmed getting help?
10. How are those who were harmed getting help?
11. Is the situation under control?
12. How certain are you that the situation is under control?
13. Is there any immediate danger?
14. What is being done in response to what happened?
15. Who is in charge?
16. What can we expect next?
17. What are you advising people to do? What can people do to protect themselves and their families – now and in the future – from harm?
18. How long will it be before the situation returns to normal?
19. What help has been requested or offered from others?
20. What responses have you received?
21. Can you be specific about the types of harm that occurred?
22. What are the names, ages and hometowns of those that were harmed?
23. Can we talk to them?
24. How much damage occurred?
25. What other damage may have occurred?
26. How certain are you about the damage?
27. How much damage do you expect?
28. What are you doing now?
29. Who else is involved in the response?
30. Why did this happen?
31. What was the cause?
32. Did you have any forewarning that this might happen?
33. Why wasn't this prevented from happening? Could this have been avoided?
34. How could this have been avoided?
35. What else can go wrong?
36. If you are not sure of the cause, what is your best guess?
37. Who caused this to happen?
38. Who is to blame?
39. Do you think those involved handled the situation well enough? What more could or should those who handled the situation have done?
40. When did your response to this begin?
41. When were you notified that something had happened?
42. Did you and other organizations disclose information promptly? Have you and other organizations been transparent?
43. Who is conducting the investigation? Will the outcome be reported to the public?
44. What are you going to do after the investigation?
45. What have you found out so far?
46. Why was more not done to prevent this from happening?
47. What is your personal opinion?
48. What are you telling your own family?
49. Are all those involved in agreement?
50. Are people over-reacting?
51. Which laws are applicable?
52. Has anyone broken the law?

## STEP 1: Assess media needs, media constraints, and internal media-relations capabilities

### 77 MOST FREQUENTLY ASKED QUESTIONS BY JOURNALISTS IN AN EMERGENCY – CONTINUED –

53. How certain are you about whether laws have been broken?
54. Has anyone made mistakes?
55. How certain are you that mistakes have not been made?
56. Have you told us everything you know?
57. What are you not telling us?
58. What effects will this have on the people involved?
59. What precautionary measures were taken?
60. Do you accept responsibility for what happened?
61. Has this ever happened before?
62. Can this happen elsewhere?
63. What is the worst-case scenario?
64. What lessons were learned?
65. Were those lessons implemented? Are they being implemented now?
66. What can be done now to prevent this from happening again? What steps need to be taken to avoid a similar event?
67. What would you like to say to those who have been harmed and to their families?
68. Is there any continuing danger?
69. Are people out of danger? Are people safe?
70. Will there be inconvenience to employees or to the public? What can people do to help?
71. How much will all this cost?
72. Are you able and willing to pay the costs?
73. Who else will pay the costs?
74. When will we find out more?
75. What steps need to be taken to avoid a similar event? Have these steps already been taken? If not, why not?
76. Why should we trust you?
77. What does this all mean?

STEP 1: Assess media needs, media constraints, and internal media-relations capabilities

## IV. What types of stories typically attract the largest audiences and gain the highest ratings?

- disasters or other high-profile events;
- high personal drama;
- heroism;
- first-time events;
- extraordinary achievements;
- extraordinary failures;
- new diseases;
- controversy or conflict;
- malpractice and negligence;
- large amount of money – made or lost;
- scandals;
- many people adversely affected;
- children adversely affected;
- situations that appear to be out of control;
- unexpected events;
- rapid or surprising expansion of adverse effects (the "ripple effect");
- polarity of views;
- miracles; and
- villains, victims and heroes.

## V. What do news editors and producers typically want from news sources?

- accurate and truthful information;
- evidence-based information;
- regular updates;
- early disclosure of information;
- brief, concise and succinct information;
- transparency;
- passion;
- first-hand information (for example, what did you see?);
- information with a different slant than information reported by other media outlets;
- graphics and visual information (for example, photographs, pictures, charts, timelines, diagrams, flowcharts, maps, drawings, videos and animations) in formats the media can easily use;
- simple statistics – with explanations if possible;
- flowcharts, figures or outlines for complicated issues, especially anything complex involving numbers;
- context (part of a wider picture) comments or explanation from the highest authority possible;
- information on economic costs;
- controversy;
- expertise;
- balanced information;
- human interest;
- timely cooperation and access to people, places and information;
- an engaging, dynamic or unusual personality;
- celebrity status; and
- respect for media deadlines.

# 1.2: ASSESS THE CONSTRAINTS OF THE MEDIA

There are a host of organizational, legal and professional constraints that affect the ability of journalists to become informed and to cover a story effectively. Each of the following constraints must be recognized and addressed when developing media communication plans and preparing for media interviews.

## I. Media constraints

### 1. Diversity

The media are not monolithic. There is a wide variety in media types (for example, broadcast, print and online); in their markets and market size; and in the practices and tasks carried out within organizations (for example, editorials, headline writing, reporting, columns and opinion pieces).

### 2. Subject-matter expertise

Many journalists lack subject-matter expertise in medicine, statistics and the health sciences. They are, however, experts in gathering, interpreting and reporting news.

### 3. Resources

Many media organizations do not have the resources needed to prepare, in advance, background information (such as graphics and videotape) on potential emergencies. In addition, news organizations seldom have the resources needed to maintain offices and reporters in distant sites. As a result, it is often difficult getting reporters and equipment to the site of an emergency.

### 4. Generalists

Most journalists are generalists rather than specialists, even in large media organizations. Journalists are often shuffled among content areas ("beats"). This shuffling provides staffing flexibility for management and is especially important when there are few staff journalists. During an emergency, the story could be assigned to any available reporter. This can result in journalists assigned to cover a public health emergency with little experience, background or specialized knowledge.

### 5. Skills

One of the most admired skills of professional journalists is their ability to quickly "get the story" on almost any topic and to report the event in an accurate, engaging and balanced manner. The ideal journalist knows how to gather information quickly (thus meeting deadlines), how to nurture sources (thus ensuring a steady flow of information), and how to report the news "objectively" (thus not alienating sources, compromising credibility, or driving away audiences). The common approach to objectivity is to cite multiple sources reflecting diverse, even opposing, viewpoints that may or may not be well-informed or meet scientific standards of evidence.

### 6. Career advancement

Journalists often advance in their careers by moving from smaller media markets to larger media markets. One result of this is high staff turnover. Therefore the assigned journalist may be unfamiliar with the community and with the public health, public safety and emergency management officials who serve that community. By the time journalists develop close working relationships with these officials they may find that they are ready to move to a new job.

## 7. Watchdogs

Many journalists perceive themselves as "watchdogs" of government and industry. They therefore expect transparency in decision-making. They are often suspicious if access to information is denied or if answers to questions are not forthcoming. They may probe for underlying political, economic or personal motives. However, this perceived watchdog role varies across different types and sizes of media and is often issue-specific.

## 8. Scepticism

Many journalists are wary of developing close professional relationships with government or industry officials. In an attempt to balance their role as watchdogs, journalists may feel a professional obligation to adopt a critical and sceptical stance regarding the activities of government and industry. This attitude, however, is often less pronounced during an emergency.

## 9. Information flow and source dependency

Journalists are highly dependent upon individuals and organizations (including government officials, agencies and nongovernmental organizations) for a steady and reliable flow of newsworthy information. This flow of information makes news production more predictable, efficient and profitable. When this flow is blocked (for example, when traditional news sources are unavailable for comment or do not respond within the journalist's deadline), journalists are more likely to seek other sources, which may be less authoritative, accurate, responsible or reliable.

## 10. Source selection

Journalists tend to rely on certain types of sources more than others. These choices largely depend on perceptions of trustworthiness and accessibility. Sources relied upon more include medical personnel, academics and scientists.

## 11. Newsworthiness

When covering health and medical controversies, journalists frequently focus on underlying political or social conflict rather than on the science itself. Controversy and conflict are often easier to cover than the details of complex issues.

## 12. Uncertainty

Journalists vary greatly in how they respond to admissions of uncertainty. Some journalists view early acknowledgements of uncertainty as an indicator of trustworthiness and transparency. Others have a more negative view of the cautious and hedging language of scientific and medical experts. As a result, they may seek out less reputable or less well-informed sources who are willing to speak out on an issue with greater certainty and with less caution, even though that certainty may be unfounded.

## 13. Legal constraints

Journalists are less constrained than public health officials by legal requirements designed to protect citizen privacy and personal information. For example, journalists will often ask public health officials for the names and addresses of victims before family members have been notified. This constraint is a frequent source of tension between health officials and journalists who cover health-related issues and emergencies. Public heath officials and journalists often struggle with the issue of how best to balance transparency with the right to privacy.

## 14. Special populations

Journalists are often ill equipped to meet the information needs of special populations during health-related emergencies. They also may not see it as their job or role to communicate directly with these audiences. Special populations include elderly people, disabled people, homeless people, housebound populations, racial and cultural minorities, linguistic minorities, illiterate populations, transient populations (for example, tourists, business travellers and migrant workers) and institutionalized populations. Because mass media outlets tailor their content to reach particular demographic groups, it is the role of the public health body to get its message to as many different audiences through as many different channels as possible. This includes special audiences who cannot or will not receive, understand or act upon the public health message.

## 15. Competition

Competition within and among media organizations (as well as among journalists) is often intense, especially in larger media markets. Many news organizations compete zealously against one another for viewers, listeners or readers. Much of this competition is centred around getting the story out first, or reporting information that competitors do not have. Competition is a major source of media sensationalism and inaccuracy.

## 16. Deadlines

Journalists assign an extremely high priority to meeting deadlines and almost all face the relentless pace of daily deadlines. This pace is even greater for 24-hour a day news media. Sources that make journalists miss their deadlines are generally looked upon with disfavour and may be bypassed in the future. Public health officials and journalists often struggle with the issue of how best to balance the competing demands associated with deadlines with the need for more time to gather information.

# 1.3: ASSESS INTERNAL MEDIA-RELATIONS CAPABILITIES

Quick response capabilities are crucial to establishing an organization as the primary source of information for the media during an emergency. To assess an organization's internal media-relations capabilities, an assessment tool such as the one shown in **BOX 1.2** should be used. The list should be adapted to meet local needs and should be as comprehensive as possible.

> **BOX 1.2: INTERNAL MEDIA-RELATIONS CAPABILITIES – AN ASSESSMENT TOOL**
>
> 1. The organization should have a written plan and documented procedures for interacting with the media during an emergency.
> 2. The organization should have:
>    - an agency staff member and at least one alternate assigned the role and responsibilities of a public information officer in an emergency;
>    - a written document that clearly identifies lines of authority and responsibilities for the public information officer and the media communication team during an emergency; and
>    - a workplan and relief scheduling plan for a media communication team to maintain 24-hour a day operations, two to three work shifts a day, for several days, weeks or possibly months.
> 3. The organization should have the following in place:
>    - procedures for verification of the accuracy of messages;
>    - procedures for clearance of information released to the media, partners and the public;
>    - procedures for coordinating with partner organizations to ensure message timeliness, accuracy and consistency; and
>    - procedures for liaison between the organization and an emergency operations centre (EOC).
> 4. The organization should have information kits for reporters prepared in advance that include contact information directories, informational materials, policies, checklists and manuals.
> 5. The organization should have the following in place:
>    - procedures for routing all media calls to the public information officer during an emergency;
>    - procedures for responding to routine media requests for information;
>    - procedures for triaging media enquiries if requests for information exceed the capacity of the agency;
>    - procedures for when, where and how to hold a news conference;
>    - procedures for releasing media advisories, news releases and fact-sheets;
>    - procedures for monitoring news coverage (for example, to determine messages needed, misinformation to be corrected, and levels of media interest and concern); and
>    - procedures for creating situation reports.
> 6. The organization should have a plan for communicating directly to the public and key stakeholders, including a plan to:
>    - set up and staff a specialized telephone information service (or "hotline") for the public, reporters, clinicians or other key stakeholders during an emergency;
>    - set up specialized web sites;
>    - monitor public concerns to determine the messages needed;
>    - monitor misinformation that needs to be corrected;
>    - monitor levels of public concern;
>    - monitor levels of employee interest and concern;
>    - ensure the accuracy, timeliness, regular updating and relevance of web site information;
>    - monitor information on other web sites; and
>    - publicize organization contact information.

## INTERNAL MEDIA-RELATIONS CAPABILITIES – AN ASSESSMENT TOOL – CONTINUED –

7. The organization should have a plan for coordinating communications with partner organizations, including a plan to:
   - respond to requests and enquiries from partners and special interest groups;
   - hold briefings for and with partner organizations;
   - translate situation reports, health alerts and meeting notes into information appropriate for partners;
   - log calls from legislators and special interest groups; and
   - set up dedicated communication lines for key partners (for example, police, elected officials, fire departments and hospitals).
8. The organization should have a directory of 24 hours a day 7 days a week contact information for media personnel and public information officers from partner organizations.
9. The organization should have plans for holding community meetings, small group briefings and other face-to-face meetings as appropriate.
10. The organization should periodically assess the media-relations training needs of its own staff and participate with other organizations to assess the media-relations training needs of its partners.
11. The organization should have a designated lead spokesperson (plus back up) for various emergency scenarios.
12. The organization should evaluate its desire, need and ability to use the following means to supplement communications through newspapers, television and radio:
    - posters;
    - web sites;
    - toll-free telephone lines;
    - public meetings;
    - email list;
    - text messaging and other mobile telephone messaging services;
    - broadcast fax;
    - letters by mail;
    - newsletters;
    - submissions to partner newsletters;
    - regular or special partner conference calls;
    - door-to-door canvassing;
    - information inserts in public utility bill mailings;
    - community bulletin boards;
    - library bulletin boards;
    - post offices bulletin boards;
    - community civil defence networks;
    - government access channels (for example, on cable television);
    - mass distribution through partners (for example, churches, retailers and restaurants);
    - reverse emergency call (for example, 911) messaging; and
    - local health alert network.
13. The organization should be able to design, develop and produce materials tailored to local needs or draw on the production capabilities of local organizations.
14. The organization should evaluate the need for the following communications personnel:
    - public affairs specialist;
    - web site designer;
    - health educators;
    - audiovisual specialist;
    - graphics illustrator/artist; and
    - translators.

### INTERNAL MEDIA-RELATIONS CAPABILITIES – AN ASSESSMENT TOOL – CONTINUED –

15. The organization should evaluate the need to develop the following in advance:
    - topical fact sheets (for example, descriptions of diseases and treatment information);
    - addenda to topical fact sheets on where to obtain additional information;
    - fact sheets on the organization (with roles, responsibilities and resources);
    - lists of frequently asked questions (FAQs) for various emergency scenarios;
    - fact sheets offering advice to emergency responders, employees, families and friends of victims, parents, health care personnel, and other relevant groups on handling post-traumatic stress and media enquiries;
    - listings of experts and web links containing information on various public health emergency topics;
    - facts sheets containing recommendations for those affected;
    - scripts for telephone operators in multiple languages for various emergency scenarios;
    - holding statements (messages prepared in advance) for various emergency scenarios;
    - news-release templates for various emergency scenarios;
    - training videos; and
    - slide presentations on various emergency scenarios.
16. The organization should have plans for addressing the communication needs of special populations (for example, the elderly, immigrant populations, transient and institutionalized populations).
17. The organization should identify the most effective tools for disseminating information.
18. The organization should have a plan for evaluating, testing and revising the media communication plan.

### INFORMATION POINT: Questions to ask as part of assessing internal media-relations capabilities before, during and after an emergency

- Who is responsible for the provision of information to the public, stakeholders and partners?
  - about the overall emergency?
  - about specific issues?
- Have key messages and strategies been developed?
- What process will be used to approve messages?
- Who has the final say in what will or will not be said to the media?
- Which media communication outlets will be used?
- Who are the identified recipients (target audience) of the messages?
- Which messages will go to what media outlets (for example, detailed instructions to print media outlets and breaking news to broadcast media outlets)?
- How will media communication effectiveness be monitored and evaluated?

# STEP 2
## Develop goals, plans and strategies

**2.1:** *Develop* media communication goals and objectives

**2.2:** *Develop* a written media communication plan

**2.3:** *Develop* a partner and stakeholder strategy

# STEP 2
## Develop goals, plans and strategies

**2.1:** *Develop* media communication goals and objectives

**2.2:** *Develop* a written media communication plan

**2.3:** *Develop* a partner and stakeholder strategy

# 2.1: DEVELOP MEDIA COMMUNICATION GOALS AND OBJECTIVES

## I. Goals

At the general level, the goals of effective media communication include:

- building, maintaining or restoring trust and credibility;
- improving knowledge and understanding of the event;
- guiding and encouraging appropriate attitudes, decisions, actions and behaviours;
- avoiding unnecessary damage to the economy and minimizing political unrest;
- encouraging collaboration and cooperation;
- proactively framing the story rather than waiting until others have defined the story and then reacting;
- establishing an agency as the main source of information and expertise;
- establishing the agency as the lead authority in charge, even under conditions of uncertainty;
- easing public anxiety;
- establishing ongoing connection with the public through the media;
- gaining support for policies and plans;
- ensuring informed decision-making;
- addressing rumours and misinformation;
- encouraging appropriate behaviours;
- encouraging constructive dialogue among stakeholders;
- engaging the public; and
- reducing the threat of panic.

### BOX 2.1: PANIC AVOIDANCE AS A GOAL

Many communication plans list the avoidance of panic as a major goal. Panic describes an intense contagious fear causing individuals to think only of themselves.

**Risk factors for panic include:**

- the belief that there is only a small chance of escape;
- the perception that there are no accessible escape routes;
- perceiving oneself at high risk of being seriously injured or killed;
- available but limited resources for assistance;
- perceptions of a "first come, first served" system;
- a perceived lack of effective management of the event;
- a perceived lack of control;
- crowd ("mob") psychology and dynamics; and
- authorities that have lost their credibility.

However, studies indicate that panic is rare, and that most people respond cooperatively and adaptively to natural and man-made disasters. Panic avoidance should never be used as a rationale for false reassurance or for lack of transparency on the part of authorities.

Panic may be more likely following a bio-terrorism attack involving contagious, dreaded or lethal diseases such as plague or smallpox. In such cases, a crucial factor in determining the public response will be the presence, actions and words of respected, credible authorities.

In the specific case of emergency events, the major informational goals should be adapted to meet local needs, but would typically include:

- providing accurate, relevant, timely, transparent, understandable, consistent and credible information about the event;
- informing and educating the public, public health practitioners, community leaders, the media and other interested or affected parties prior to the event so they are better prepared to respond;
- avoiding panic (**BOX 2.1**);
- establishing and maintaining appropriate levels of public vigilance and concern;
- addressing rumours, inaccuracies and misperceptions through early and frequent reporting of information;
- establishing or maintaining public confidence in the ability of authorities to respond to and manage the event; and
- informing people of how to mitigate the effects of an emergency.

**BOX 2.2** provides an example of a media communication goal statement during an emergency event. The statement has been adapted from an actual public health department document relating to an outbreak of West Nile virus. As always such goals should be adapted to specific local circumstances and needs.

> **BOX 2.2: EXAMPLE OF A MEDIA COMMUNICATION GOAL STATEMENT**
>
> The goals of the agency in the event of a disease outbreak are to:
> - maintain, increase or restore trust as an overriding goal;
> - inform and educate governmental authorities, municipal officials, the public and the media regarding:
>   - details of the outbreak
>   - outbreak prevention measures, including personal protection measures
>   - the agency's surveillance plan
>   - the agency's response plan
>   - disease control methods;
> - increase awareness of the disease, its transmission, its prevention and its diagnosis among health care providers, including general and hospital practitioners;
> - increase awareness among health care providers of the use of control measures;
> - communicate disease control information and recommendations to governmental authorities, municipal officials, the public and media in a timely and efficient manner; and
> - collaborate and cooperate with key partners and nongovernmental organizations to review and disseminate communication materials.

## II. Objectives

The major distinction between goals and objectives is that a goal describes a desired end state while objectives describe measurable steps to achieve this – objectives should therefore be:

**S**pecific
**M**easurable
**A**ssignable
**R**easonable
**T**ime-related.

An example of an objective would be the percentage of the target audience that by a set time:

- has heard the public health message;
- has taken a recommended public health action; and
- has made changes in attitude or behaviour because of a public health communication.

## 2.2: DEVELOP A WRITTEN MEDIA COMMUNICATION PLAN

Effective media communication requires a written media communication plan prepared and endorsed by senior management in advance (**BOX 2.3**). Such a plan allows for a proactive, quick and effective response during an emergency since many of the necessary communication decisions and activities will have already been decided upon. If carefully designed, a media communication plan can save precious time when an emergency occurs and can enable leaders and spokespersons to focus on the quality, accuracy and speed of their response. Once completed, the communication plan should be evaluated, revised and updated regularly.

A key component of any effective media communication plan will be the identification of:

- contingency plans for emergency scenarios;
- background materials for emergency scenarios, as well as draft or template news releases;
- lead spokespersons and public information officers adequately trained in communication and public health;
- procedures for gathering information on what has happened so far, what is currently happening, and what is expected to happen;
- training requirements and obligations for members of the media communication team;
- preferred channels of communication – for example, through news releases, news conferences, the internet, a toll-free telephone line, brochures, radio announcements, special events, door-to-door canvassing or media interviews;
- target audiences;
- goals – for example, in informing, persuading or motivating;
- communication tasks to be accomplished, and who is responsible;
- specific, measurable, assignable, reasonable and time-related objectives focused on specific targeted audiences;
- all those inside and outside the organization who should be contacted and informed when an emergency occurs;
- contact information for the lead spokesperson and public information officer of partner agencies (**FIGURE TWO**);
- partners and their available resources;
- emergency contact lists with clearly marked responsibilities;
- procedures for ensuring contact lists are regularly checked and updated;
- well-publicized agency polices and procedures regarding employee contacts with the media;
- a time-line showing the start and completion of each phase of the media communication plan;
- directions on where copies of the communication plan can be obtained;
- means for measuring achievement of the plan's objectives; and
- means for early intervention if messages are not getting across or if communication objectives are not being met.

## BOX 2.3: BASIC INFORMATION TYPICALLY INCLUDED IN A MEDIA COMMUNICATION PLAN

**A media communications plan should:**

- describe and designate staff roles and responsibilities for different emergency scenarios;
- designate who is accountable for leading the response;
- designate who is responsible for implementing various actions;
- designate who needs to be consulted during the process;
- designate who needs to be informed about what is taking place;
- designate who will be the lead spokesperson and backup for different scenarios;
- include procedures for information verification, clearance and approval;
- include procedures for coordinating with important stakeholders and partners (for example, with other health agencies, and law enforcement and elected officials);
- include procedures to secure the required human, financial, logistical and physical support and resources (such as people, space, equipment and food) for media communication operations during a short, medium and prolonged public health event (24 hours a day 7 days a week if needed);
- include agreements on releasing information and on ownership (who releases what, when and how);
- include polices and procedures regarding employee contacts from the media;
- outline well thought out contingency plans for various scenarios;
- include regularly checked and updated media contact lists (including after-hours news desks);
- include regularly checked and updated partner contact lists (day and night);
- outline exercises and drills for testing the media communication plan as part of larger preparedness and response training;
- identify subject-matter experts (for example, university professors) willing to collaborate during an emergency, and develop and test contact lists (day and night); know their perspectives in advance;
- identify target audiences;
- identify preferred communication channels (for example, telephone hotlines, radio announcements, news conferences, web site updates and faxes) to communicate with the public, key stakeholders and partners;
- contain holding statements (messages prepared in advance), core messages and message templates;
- contain fact sheets, question-and-answer sheets, talking points and other supplementary materials for potential scenarios;
- contain a signed endorsement of the media communication plan from the agency's director;
- contain procedures for posting/updating information on a web site;
- contain task checklists for the first 2, 4, 8, 12,16, 24 and 48 hours; and
- contain procedures for evaluating, revising and updating the media communication plan on a regular basis.

## FIGURE TWO: WORKSHEET FOR IDENTIFYING ORGANIZATIONS AND INDIVIDUALS TO BE CONTACTED DURING AN EMERGENCY

| Group | Notifications (check those that apply) | Contact | Tel/fax day/night |
|---|---|---|---|
| Local government | Local health officer | | |
| | Local health department public information officer | | |
| | Local government officials | | |
| | Local government public information officer | | |
| | Local emergency response organizations (for example, fire, police, emergency management services and law enforcement) | | |
| | Local emergency response organization public information officers | | |
| | Local hospitals | | |
| | Other | | |
| Regional government | Regional health director | | |
| | Regional health department public information officer | | |
| | Regional government executive office | | |
| | Other regional government officials | | |
| | Other | | |
| National government | National health director | | |
| | National health director public information officer | | |
| | National government executive office | | |
| | Other national government officials | | |
| | Other | | |
| International organizations | WHO regional office | | |
| | WHO country office | | |
| | Other international organizations | | |
| | Nongovernmental organizations | | |
| | Other | | |
| Local, regional, national and international media organizations | | | |
| | | | |
| | | | |
| | | | |
| | | | |
| | | | |
| Other partner and stakeholder organizations (for example, experts at local universities and in the scientific community) | | | |
| | | | |
| | | | |
| | | | |
| | | | |
| | | | |
| | | | |
| | | | |
| | | | |
| Others | | | |
| | | | |
| | | | |
| | | | |
| | | | |
| | | | |

# I. Media communication during an emergency

During a major emergency, health departments may receive hundreds or even thousands of enquiries each day from the media, the public, partner organizations and other interested parties. Dealing with these enquiries must be properly and systematically planned and managed if timely responses are to be provided. One device for accomplishing this is to organize media communication efforts during an emergency according to predetermined task areas, with teams assigned to cover one or more of these areas. Many of the specific tasks listed below are routinely carried out during normal times – the difference between emergency and non-emergency communication is often one of staffing and workload in each of the following task areas:

- media communications leadership;
- media relations;
- message and materials development;
- partner and stakeholder outreach;
- web sites;
- administrative and technical support;
- studio and broadcast;
- research and media monitoring;
- hotlines;
- community health education;
- workforce communications;
- clinician communications;
- policy-maker and legislative communications; and
- information management.

Each of these tasks is discussed in detail below.

## 1. Media communications leadership

- prepare and distribute the written media communication plan;
- activate and implement the plan after careful assessment of the situation;
- meet with agency leadership shortly after the emergency notification to discuss communication strategies and activities;
- ensure that the position of the lead spokesperson is appropriate to the scale of the emergency (for example, in a large-scale emergency, the lead spokesperson would typically be the agency head or a senior deputy);
- ensure all relevant individuals and offices have copies of the media communication plan;
- ensure all relevant individuals and offices have been trained in how to implement the plan;
- bring in the required resources – human and logistical – as specified in the plan;
- assemble the communication team shortly after notification, brief them on the event, consult with them on what needs to be communicated, and delegate tasks and assignments;
- contact other responding organizations to learn what steps they are planning to take;
- disseminate predetermined guidance on information verification, clearance and approval;
- contact and confirm the availability of predetermined lead spokespersons;
- review the strengths, weaknesses and training of lead spokespersons;
- brief the lead spokespersons and review their responsibilities with them;
- inform all employees who will serve as the agency lead spokespersons in the emergency;
- remind all employees of agency policies regarding contact with the media;

- ensure notification of those on the predetermined list of people inside and outside the organization who are to be informed when an emergency occurs and what the organization's response is or will be – given the importance of this, consider assigning a staff member to maintaining the list and confirming that notification has occurred;
- ensure coordination and dissemination of information with other agencies before release;
- balance the need to coordinate the dissemination of information with other agencies with the need to engage in prompt and timely disclosure;
- provide periodic briefings on event status and strategies with agency leaders;
- provide periodic briefings on event status and strategies with the media communication team that cover:
  - what is known
  - what is not known
  - what is being done
  - what is being recommended;
- provide periodic briefings on event status and strategies with select stakeholders;
- conduct news briefings;
- implement the predetermined strategy for coordinating internal and external communication activities;
- determine operational hours for emergency communication activities, including shift changes;
- be aware of (and respond appropriately to) signs of stress among staff (including oneself); and
- carry out all leadership responsibilities and tasks in a calm and professional manner.

## 2. Media relations

- organize and conduct news briefings (based on media deadlines when possible);
- produce and distribute timely news releases and other media materials;
- respond to media requests and enquiries;
- provide support for spokespersons; and
- coordinate responses to media enquiries.

## 3. Message and materials development

- develop and distribute draft talking and/or message points and message maps (see section **4.2**);
- activate predetermined procedures for information verification, approval and clearance;
- create drafts of news releases, fact sheets, questions-and-answer sheets (Q&As), frequently asked questions (FAQs), speeches, video scripts, public service announcements and other communication materials;
- create appropriate graphics and other visual material to support messages and other communication approaches;
- ensure that information contained in communication materials is accurate, current and cleared for release; and
- ensure coordination and consistency of messages internally and across other responding organizations.

## 4. Partner and stakeholder outreach

- maintain open channels of communication with partners and stakeholders in interested or affected governmental, nongovernmental, not-for-profit and private-sector organizations; and
- coordinate announcements and release of information with partner organizations.

## 5. Web site

- open predetermined web page templates for use on the organization's web site;
- establish and maintain links to other web sites;
- post information about the event on the web site;
- oversee the prompt updating of materials on the web site;
- develop (as required) password-protected web sites to share information within the organization and among partners;
- determine who needs to approve the posting and updating of information on the web site; and
- assess internet/web site visits, hits and usage.

## 6. Administrative and technical support

- manage essential administrative and technical tasks; and
- distribute communication materials.

## 7. Studio and broadcast

- activate equipment and support the broadcasting of news conferences and other media events; and
- record and log all news conferences and briefings.

## 8. Research and media monitoring

- analyse feedback from other communication teams for patterns and cross-cutting trends;
- prioritize media outlets for scanning and monitoring based on where the target audience goes for information;
- scan print and broadcast media for information that could help or hinder the response effort;
- scan web sites for information that could help or hinder the response effort;
- scan all other media outlets for information that could help or hinder the response effort;
- scan, collect and analyse data (for example, from public polls or focus groups) on audience knowledge, attitudes and behaviour regarding the issue or event; and
- provide feedback on scanning and monitoring activities to other emergency communication team members.

## 9. Hotlines

- respond to hotline requests for information from the public and the media;
- depending upon the number of enquiries, consider establishing separate hotlines for the media, the public, policy-makers and other key stakeholders;
- distribute requests for information from the media, the public and other stakeholders to the appropriate person or organization;
- provide feedback from the hotline calls to other emergency communication team members; and
- coordinate the use of the hotline with other responding organizations.

## 10. Community health education

- develop and ensure distribution of health education information to interested or affected communities and special populations through appropriate media outlets;
- identify public health education needs through media monitoring activities and feedback from partner organizations;
- facilitate meetings with interested or affected communities or special populations; and
- develop public information campaign materials if needed.

## 11. Workforce communications

- identify and open predetermined channels for communicating with the public health workforce, including public health professionals;
- work with other team members on message development and dissemination;
- arrange for regular briefings of the workforce;
- coordinate information dissemination efforts with other teams; and
- provide feedback from the workforce to other emergency communication team members.

## 12. Clinician communications

- identify and open predetermined channels for communicating with clinicians;
- coordinate with other programme networks for clinician message dissemination;
- arrange and conduct regular briefings for clinician networks;
- respond to requests and enquiries from clinicians and clinician groups; and
- provide feedback from clinicians to other emergency communication team members.

## 13. Policy-maker and legislative communications

- identify and open predetermined channels for communicating with policy-makers;
- distribute communication materials and updates to elected officials, legislators and special interest groups;
- respond to requests from elected officials, legislators and special interest groups;
- arrange routine briefings for selected policy-makers;
- work with other team members to evaluate materials for policy-makers; and
- provide feedback from policy-makers to other emergency communication team members.

## 14. Information management

- collect, review and finalize event informational materials;
- maintain a database and/or log of event information and materials;
- facilitate clearance and approval of printed communication materials;
- create a central repository of communication materials; and
- create an efficient system for the retrieval and distribution of communication materials.

## 2.3: DEVELOP A PARTNER AND STAKEHOLDER STRATEGY

In many types of emergencies, public health will be integrated into a larger emergency response system. Public health is thus likely to share leadership with a wide range of governmental and nongovernmental partners, including law enforcement, fire departments, hospitals, emergency medical services, crisis managers, the military and intelligence agencies. Cooperation with partners is a crucial part of effective media communication as they can:

- access specialized and needed information that could not otherwise be obtained;
- provide specific or alternative points of view based on their expertise and location;
- provide supplemental resources (such as human, financial, logistical and physical) that cannot otherwise be accessed;
- validate and endorse messages; and
- serve liaison or intermediary roles with important stakeholders.

Potential partners will also bring their own focus, competencies, personality traits and organizational culture (**BOX 2.4**) that will impact upon how and what they try to communicate. In general, however, successful partnering will help to display unity, improve the chance of coordinated effort, enhance preparedness prior to the event and reinforce the public perception of trust. Such partnering is typically most effective when differences are resolved or harmonized in advance, when messages are consistent across partner organizations and where there is a contingency plan for situations where partners cannot agree.

As a central element in any media communication plan, proactive efforts should be made to establish working relationships with the media before an emergency occurs (**BOX 2.5**). Effective communication responses to public health emergencies are built on such pre-established relationships with the media. During a public health emergency, other potential partners include anyone or any organization with a strategic role to perform, including:

- government agencies (local, provincial, national and international);
- international organizations;
- nongovernmental organizations (NGOs);
- private-volunteer organizations (PVOs);
- military organizations;
- police departments and other law enforcement agencies;
- fire departments;
- hospitals;
- animal health agencies;
- elected and appointed officials;
- legislative offices;
- relief agencies;
- transportation organizations;
- educational organizations;
- religious organizations;
- business organizations;
- mental health organizations;
- electricity companies;
- water authorities; and
- telephone companies.

## STEP 2: Develop goals, plans and strategies

### BOX 2.4: ELEMENTS OF ORGANIZATIONAL CULTURE

- basic organizational beliefs and shared values;
- attitudes and beliefs regarding openness and trust;
- history of the organization, including folklore and stories about past events;
- leadership styles;
- lines of communication, including protocols regarding the communication of ideas;
- task commitment;
- reward system;
- teamwork and cooperation;
- structure and organization of work;
- motivation;
- expectations (for example, "providing a high level of service with a minimum of resources");
- recruitment (including selection bias);
- education and training;
- attitudes towards technology (high-tech or low-tech);
- appearance, fitness and demeanour;
- individual initiative; and
- credo (for example, "the patient always comes first"; "leave no one behind"; or "put the needs of the organization above your own").

### BOX 2.5: ESTABLISHING WORKING RELATIONSHIPS WITH THE MEDIA BEFORE AN EMERGENCY OCCURS

**Outreach efforts should include:**

- identifying and meeting with reporters and editors who cover your organization;
- exchanging contact information with media organizations (telephone, fax and email);
- arranging ad hoc or periodic meetings with editorial boards;
- holding roundtable discussions to receive feedback from reporters or editors;
- holding briefing sessions to share information about your organization; and
- inviting reporters to participate in preparedness drills and training exercises.

**Before pursuing these activities:**

- determine your goals – for example, better communication, better relationships or better reporting;
- determine your specific objectives – for example:
  - obtaining feedback from reporters on your performance – both generally and issue-specific ("How are we doing"? "How could we improve"? "How can we work together better in the future"?)
  - improving reporters' knowledge of your organization's plans and procedures for responding to an emergency
  - informing reporters on important public health concepts, issues and topics, such as disease characteristics; infectious disease control procedures; toxicology and epidemiology; agents that might be used by terrorists (for example, biological, chemical, explosive and radiological); risk communication; incident command systems; the legal constraints on public health policy and practice; and guidelines for reporters on how to protect themselves, their crews and their equipment during a public health emergency;
- share your media communication goals and objectives with others in your organization – get feedback;
- determine which media (for example, local, provincial, regional or national) to include in your outreach efforts;
- recognize that media outreach efforts now may or may not produce more favourable news coverage by reporters; and
- expect no favours.

STEP 2: Develop goals, plans and strategies

> **INFORMATION POINT: Considerations when developing relationships with partners**
> - Which partners are most important for each type of emergency situation (for example, infectious disease outbreaks in human or animal populations, bio-terrorism, chemical explosions, nuclear and radiological events or natural disasters)?
> - What issues are most important to the partner organization?
> - How can the partner organization contribute and help?
> - What resources can the partner organization bring?
> - What are the partner organization's strengths and weaknesses?
> - What credibility does the partner organization bring to the situation?
> - Will the partner organization commit to collaborating in and coordinating message development?
> - Will the partner organization commit to the joint release of information?
> - How will joint statements be issued?
> - What message clearance and approval process will be followed?
> - Who will be the point of contact in the partner organization?
> - What is the overall nature of the existing relationship? For example, is it currently:
>   - apathetic
>   - neutral
>   - supportive
>   - non-supportive
>   - critical
>   - adversarial
>   - ambivalent?
> - What specific issues are likely to be points of agreement or disagreement?
> - What are the partner organization's expectations in an emergency (for example, in regards to level of involvement)?

> **INFORMATION POINT: Common mistakes in working with partners**
> - lack of listening, caring and empathy;
> - inadequate access;
> - inadequate relationship building prior to an emergency;
> - lack of clarity in messages;
> - lack of dedication and commitment;
> - lack of respect for core values and protocols;
> - lack of resources;
> - misreading of strengths and weaknesses;
> - perceptions of arrogance;
> - misreading the credibility brought to the situation;
> - lack of consistency in messages, data and tone;
> - lack of timeliness;
> - lack of coordination and synchronization;
> - competition for visibility and publicity; and
> - not understanding needs or motivations.

**STEP 2: Develop goals, plans and strategies**

## INFORMATION POINT: Working with partners

Take the following actions to work effectively with partners before, during and after a public health emergency.

| Action to take | Explanation |
| --- | --- |
| Identify strategic partners for various scenarios before an emergency | *Know specifically who must, and who can, help during an emergency* |
| Develop a profile of the partner organization and of your counterpart in that organization | *Identify the mission, values, goals, orientation and issues important to the partner organization and to your counterpart in that organization* |
| Determine the strengths, weaknesses and potential media communication roles of the partner organization | *Analyse clearly and specifically what resources and credibility the partner organization has and is willing to add to effective media communication during an emergency* |
| Determine and coordinate your respective media communication roles and responsibilities in various emergency scenarios | *Work out the details of who, what, why, where, when and how. Determine how joint statements will be issued. Define the clearance and approval process.* |
| Develop contact sheets | *Develop, and carry with you at all times, lists of 24 hours a day 7 days a week contact information for your counterparts (and back-ups) in each partner organization* |
| Understand the organizational hierarchy of the partner organization | *Find out who makes the decisions in the partner organization and make sure you are connected to the right person for information, clearance or action* |

# STEP 3
## Train communicators

**3.1:** *Train* the media communication team
**3.2:** *Train* a public information officer
**3.3:** *Train* a designated lead spokesperson

# STEP 3
## Train communicators

**3.1:** *Train* the media communication team
**3.2:** *Train* a public information officer
**3.3:** *Train* a designated lead spokesperson

# 3.1: TRAIN THE MEDIA COMMUNICATION TEAM

Members of the media communication team should receive training in all the seven steps described in this handbook in addition to general training in public health issues. The following sample public health emergency communications training agenda could also be usefully provided to agency leaders and technical experts. If they have a better understanding of what the communication team is trying to accomplish and how team members think through communication tasks, it makes the process much smoother and more consistent. In all cases, training should be adapted in line with local practices.

## I. Sample public health emergency communications training agenda

### 1. Developing effective messages during an emergency

   a. Overview of the basic principles and tools of communication during an emergency (see **ANNEXES 9–11**):
      i. How people form risk perceptions and make risk judgements
      ii. How people process risk information in high-stress situations
      iii. How people form perceptions of trust
   b. Types of messages
   c. Developing talking points, key messages and supporting information
   d. Resources for developing effective messages
   e. Methods for testing messages

### 2. Communication pitfalls and solutions

   a. Uncertainty and/or lack of knowledge
   b. Worst-case speculation
   c. Unsubstantiated allegations, accusations or rumours
   d. Guarantees and promises
   e. Over-reassurance
   f. Lack of inclusion

### 3. Methods and means of effective communication outreach

   a. Selecting appropriate written and spoken channels for communication
   b. Working effectively with partner organizations before, during and after an emergency
   c. Planning and conducting effective meetings with stakeholders before, during and after an emergency
   d. Responding to difficult questions in group settings
   e. Choosing between alternative outreach channels
   f. Addressing special population needs
   g. Addressing diversity, and cross-cultural needs
   h. Using outside experts (third parties) to communicate agency messages
   i. Developing effective graphics and other visual materials

## 4. Verbal and non-verbal communication skills

  a. Verbal communication skills
  b. Non-verbal communication skills
  c. Selecting and training spokespersons
  d. Optimizing the effectiveness of spokespersons

## 5. Working with the media during an emergency

  a. Challenges to effective media communication
  b. Strategies for successful media interactions
  c. Skills needed for successful media interactions (such as the skills needed to bridge from one message to another)
  d. Advantages and disadvantages of different media outlets and different media formats (for example, sit-down interviews, panel discussions and radio call-in shows)
  e. Methods for handling aggressive media interviews (including ambush interviews and investigative reporters)

## 6. Conducting effective communication drills, exercises and role-playing

## 3.2: TRAIN A PUBLIC INFORMATION OFFICER

A well-trained public information officer (PIO) or the equivalent, trained in both communications and public health, is a necessary requirement for effective media communications during public health emergencies. Public information officers must either be able to serve as the lead media spokesperson for the organization, or to provide support and back up to the lead spokesperson. To achieve this they must be able to perform a variety of tasks before, during and after an emergency (**BOX 3.1**).

### BOX 3.1: MEDIA COMMUNICATION COMPETENCIES OF PUBLIC INFORMATION OFFICERS

**A public information officer should be able to:**
- describe the roles and responsibilities of a public information officer during a public health emergency;
- demonstrate skills in written and oral communication;
- communicate effectively with partner agencies involved in an emergency;
- demonstrate skills in team building, negotiation and conflict resolution;
- develop a media communication plan integrated with the overall emergency response plan of the organization;
- develop and maintain files of up-to-date informational materials and resources for various emergency scenarios (for example, fact sheets related to chemical, biological and radiological agents);
- develop and maintain staffing plans for a 24 hours a day 7 days a week response to an emergency;
- select and prioritize media outlets;
- compile media contact lists, partner contact lists and expert contact lists;
- develop and operate a multi-agency Joint Information Centre (JIC);
- access, use, interpret and display emergency-related data;
- describe basic principles for communicating effectively to the media in an emergency;
- describe the basic elements of the organization's emergency operations plan;
- train other spokespersons;
- develop, evaluate and implement media communication exercises and drills;
- operate communication equipment identified in the media communication plan (phone lines, telephone banks, computers, walkie-talkies, personal digital assistants, cameras, copiers, fax machines and radios);
- develop and deliver event-specific information to:
    - the media
    - partner organizations
    - agency staff and employees
    - other government agencies
    - nongovernmental organizations
    - the public; and
- remain calm, and convey confidence and composure under pressure.

## 3.3: TRAIN A DESIGNATED LEAD SPOKESPERSON

In almost all emergencies, a designated lead spokesperson is a necessity. The public and media tend to like and trust a familiar face and voice. The image or voice of the lead spokesperson is often the first message an organization sends out during an emergency. Having a lead spokesperson also simplifies information flow and promotes the consistency of message content. The lead spokesperson may be the organization's director or someone else identified with the leadership. In any case, the designated individual must posses the personal and professional characteristics listed in **BOX 3.2**.

> **BOX 3.2: PERSONAL AND PROFESSIONAL CHARACTERISTICS OF A DESIGNATED LEAD SPOKESPERSON**
>
> **The designated lead spokesperson should:**
> - possess excellent media skills;
> - have sufficient authority or expertise to be accepted as speaking on behalf of the organization;
> - possess or work to develop good professional relationships with important members of the media and other important partners and stakeholders;
> - be:
>   - perceived as authoritative and credible by stakeholders, partners and the public
>   - at ease with the media
>   - knowledgeable (generally and specifically) about the emergency, its dynamics and its management
>   - a subject-matter expert on the event or able to delegate to subject-matter experts
>   - resourceful; and
> - be able to:
>   - learn quickly
>   - respond to sensitive questions within their areas of expertise in a professional and sensitive manner
>   - effectively respond to hostile questions
>   - stay on message yet remain flexible and able to make decisions quickly
>   - offer examples, anecdotes and stories
>   - provide effective on-the-spot responses to media enquiries
>   - express technical knowledge or complex information in a way that can be easily understood by reporters and by the average person
>   - remain calm and composed at all times
>   - express caring, listening, empathy and compassion
>   - work well under pressure or high emotional strain
>   - accept constructive feedback
>   - share the spotlight
>   - call on the expertise of others
>   - give thanks to others and distribute praise
>   - take responsibility for things that go wrong
>   - present the appropriate tone for the audience
>   - defer, delegate and redirect questions to others as needed.

During an emergency, the lead spokesperson and other spokespersons are the public face of an organization's response. In order to deal effectively with the media during a public health emergency, the recommended approaches outlined in **BOX 3.3** should be tightly adhered to. Only those things appropriate for quotes during interviews should be expressed – there is **no such thing** as "off the record". The lead spokesperson must stay on message (i.e., avoid straying intentionally or inadvertently from the prepared key points) and be skilled in the use of bridging techniques that allow one message to be linked to another. Conversely they need to be very aware of the potential pitfalls outlined in **BOX 3.4** that must be avoided when dealing with media.

### BOX 3.3: RECOMMENDED APPROACHES FOR LEAD AND OTHER SPOKESPERSONS WHEN DEALING WITH THE MEDIA DURING AN EMERGENCY

- Listen to, acknowledge and respect the fears, anxieties and uncertainties of the public and key stakeholders.
- Remain calm and in control, even in the face of public fear, anxiety and uncertainty.
- Provide people with ways to participate, protect themselves and gain or regain a sense of personal control.
- Focus on what is known and tell reporters what follow-up actions will be taken if a question cannot be answered immediately, or tell people where to get additional information.
- Offer authentic statements and actions that communicate compassion, conviction and optimism.
- Be honest, candid, transparent, ethical, frank and open.
- Take ownership of the issue or problem.
- Remember that first impressions are lasting impressions – they matter.
- Avoid humour because it can be interpreted as uncaring or trivializing the issue.
- Be extremely careful in saying anything that could be interpreted as an unqualified absolute ("never" or "always") – it only takes one exception to disprove an absolute.
- Be the first to share bad or good news.
- Balance bad news with three or more positive, constructive or solution-oriented messages.
- Avoid mixed or inconsistent verbal and non-verbal messages.
- Be visible or readily available.
- Demonstrate media skills (verbal and non-verbal) including avoidance of major traps and pitfalls – for example, speculating about extreme worst-case scenarios, saying "there are no guarantees", repeating allegations or accusations, or saying "no comment".
- Develop and offer three concise key messages in response to each major concern.
- Continually look for opportunities to repeat the prepared key messages.
- Use clear non-technical language free of jargon and acronyms.
- Make extensive but appropriate use of visual material, personal and human-interest stories, quotes, analogies and anecdotes.
- Find out who else is being interviewed and make appropriate adjustments.
- Monitor what is being said on the internet as much as other media.
- Take the first day of an emergency very seriously – drop other obligations.
- Avoid guessing – check and double-check the accuracy of facts.
- Ensure facts offered have gone through a clearance process.
- Plan media communications programmes well in advance using the APP model (anticipate/prepare/practice) – conduct scenario planning, identify important stakeholders, anticipate questions and concerns, train spokespersons, prepare messages, test messages, anticipate follow-up questions and rehearse responses.
- Provide information on a continuous and frequent basis.
- Ensure partners (internal and external) speak with one voice.
- Have a contingency plan for when partners (internal and external) disagree.
- When possible, use research to help determine responses to messages.
- Plan public meetings carefully – unless they are carefully controlled and skilfully implemented they can backfire and result in increased public outrage and frustration.
- Encourage the use of face-to-face communication methods, including expert availability sessions, workshops and poster-based information exchanges.
- Be able to cite other credible sources of information.
- Admit when mistakes have been made – be accountable and responsible.
- Avoid attacking the credibility of those with higher perceived credibility.
- Acknowledge uncertainty.
- Seek, engage and make extensive use of support from credible third parties.

## STEP 1: Train communicators

> ### BOX 3.4: PITFALLS TO AVOID WHEN COMMUNICATING WITH THE MEDIA DURING AN EMERGENCY
>
> - **Don't assume you are the right person to be interviewed** – Negotiate with the reporter about the specific topic of the interview to ensure you are the appropriate spokesperson.
> - **Don't assume you know what the first question from the reporter will be** – Ask the reporter in advance what the first question will be. Your second answer will depend on your first answer.
> - **Don't allow the interview to stray from the topic** – Offer to cover additional topics during a separate interview. Alternatively, offer to put the reporter in touch with someone who is better able to respond than you if needed.
> - **Don't let a reporter put words in your mouth** – The reporter may use inflammatory or emotionally laden words. Do not repeat them.
> - **Don't accept a question that is improperly framed** – rephrase a question if it contains leading or loaded language, and then answer the question.
> - **Don't assume the reporter has it right** – Be on guard for claims that someone has made an allegation or has shared damaging information. Instead of reacting to such information, say: "I have not heard that" or "I would have to verify that before I could respond". Do not allow the reporter to start a fight.
> - **Don't volunteer more than you want to say** – If a reporter persists after you've answered the question, then stop. Do not answer the question again or add to your answer. Instead, wait for the next question or say: "That was my answer. Do you have another question that you would like me to address"? Say it without sarcasm, defensiveness or annoyance.
> - **Don't go "off the record"** – There is no such thing as "off the record".
> - **Don't assume your knowledge or position alone qualifies you to answer questions** – Anticipate questions. Work with your colleagues and your public information officer to anticipate as many expected questions as possible and draft the answers to as many as time permits. Nuances count. A word change here or there may make the difference to how well your answer is received. Write your first draft of the answers then edit them or have them edited. Find the key words and the bottom line – what is the point you want to make? What rings true and doesn't sound evasive?
> - **Don't go into an interview without at least three key messages** – Have prepared message points and make them at the very start of the interview. Try to get across your key message points in sound-bite format in fewer than 27 words and less than 9 seconds. Be prepared to elaborate on your prepared message points.
> - **Don't guess or fake it** – If you do not know the answer or cannot answer, say so. Give the reason why you do not know or can't answer. For example, if it's not in your area of expertise, say so.
> - **Don't speak disparagingly of others, not even in jest** – Do not assign blame either. Stick to what you know and what your organization is doing. Do not fight your battles using the media. If you do not have something nice to say, say nothing. Remind reporters that professionals often have legitimate differences of opinion.
> - **Don't buy into extreme or baseless "what if" questions** – Rephrase the question in a way that addresses the legitimate concerns of the public.
> - **Don't depend on the reporter to remember what was said** – Use a tape recorder to record sensitive interviews, if necessary. Be sure the reporter knows you are doing this before the interview.
> - **Don't ask reporters to allow you review their articles or interviews** – Offer to clarify information for them as they prepare their story. If a reporter shows you the story, understand he or she expects you to correct errors of fact not viewpoints that may differ from yours.
> - **Don't try to answer all parts of a multiple-part question** – Break down multiple-part questions and answer each part separately.
> - **Don't raise issues you do not want to see in print or on the news.**
> - **Don't say "no comment" to a reporter's question** – People often interpret "no comment" statements as showing guilt, hiding something, lying or covering up. Instead, state why you cannot answer the question. For example, say the matter is under investigation, the organization has not yet made a decision, or simply that you are not the right person to answer the question. If appropriate, indicate follow-up actions you are willing to take, including referrals or providing further information by the reporter's deadline.
> - **Don't assume you have been quoted correctly** – Have someone monitor media coverage and check whether your statements were edited incorrectly or out of context. If significant errors are discovered, seek further coverage to correct mistakes and get your points across.
> - **Don't miss the reporter's deadline** – If you miss the reporter's deadline, your perspective may go unrepresented in the reporter's story.
> - **Don't assume that facts speak for themselves or that the interview will be easy.**

# I. Tactics sometimes used to surprise or confuse a spokesperson

## 1. Sensational, negative or unrelated questions

Answer the question in as few words as possible without repeating the sensational or negative elements. Then return to one or all of the 3 key messages – recommended "bridging phrases"(see section **6.1**) to help do this include:

- *Let me emphasize again what I said before…*
- *The overall issue on the table, from my perspective, is…*
- *What's important to remember about this issue is…*
- *What I can tell you about this issue that might be helpful is…*
- *What I'm really here to discuss is the critical importance of…*
- *What all these issues boil down to is…*
- *What is really important for your readers/viewers to know is…*

## 2. Character attack

Do not attack the character of an adversary – it may be necessary to question the science, issues or goals, but not someone's character. For example, say "I can't speak for Dr X. You'll have to ask him/her. What I can address is…".

## 3. Machine-gun questioning

Be aware that a reporter might ask questions rapidly, quicken the pace, or frequently interrupt your responses. One response to this is to say "Please let me answer this question". Control the pace and take time to think.

## 4. Microphone feeding and pausing

Be aware of situations in which a good answer has been given to a controversial question, and the reporter says nothing while the cameras continue to roll. Silence on air does not make for interesting viewing unless the spokesperson is reacting nervously or uncomfortably so be aware of non-verbal cues. Avoid a "deer-in-the-headlights" appearance, fidgeting, wiping of the brow and shifting frequently in the seat. It is the reporter's job to fill the airtime so relax and wait for their next question.

## 5. Hot microphone

Assume the microphone is always on – including during "testing" and chatting **before and after** the interview.

## 6. Sensational question with an A or B dilemma

Reject both A or B if neither is valid. Explain by saying "there's actually another alternative you should consider", and give the message point. Use positive words and correct inaccuracies without repeating the negative.

## 7. Surprise prop

The reporter attempts to hand over a report, a prop, a videotape or a supposedly contaminated item (such as a glass of "contaminated" water). Avoid taking "ownership" and refuse to take or touch the item. React instead by saying, "I'm familiar with that report, and what I can say about it is…" or "I'm not familiar with that report, but what is important is…" and then go to the key message.

## II. Non-verbal communication skills

People are often highly attentive to non-verbal cues, and in high-stress emergency situations such cues can be even more important than verbal communication. In fact, non-verbal communications can provide more than 75% percent of message content, with visual information enhancing the chances that messages will be heard and understood. The exact meaning of a non-verbal communication depends upon the culture in which it occurs. For example, in Western European and American cultures non-verbal communications that are interpreted highly negatively or very positively are shown in **BOXES 3.5** and **3.6** respectively. Ways of minimizing the effect of negative non-verbal messages in general include:

- supplementing the presentation with visual aids that are easy to understand and become the focus of the presentation;
- placing visual aids, such as presentation slides, charts or a flipchart, in a central place during the presentation;
- interacting with the visual aids and with the audience;
- practising and videotaping the presentation in front of colleagues; and
- asking colleagues to critique non-verbal communication displayed in a simulated high-stress interview.

### BOX 3.5: NEGATIVELY PERCEIVED NON-VERBAL COMMUNICATION

| | |
|---|---|
| Poor eye contact | *dishonest, closed, unconcerned, nervous, lying* |
| Sitting back in chair | *not interested, unenthusiastic, unconcerned, withdrawn, distancing oneself, uncooperative* |
| Arms crossed on chest | *not interested, uncaring, not listening, arrogant, impatient, defensive, angry, stubborn, not accepting* |
| Infrequent hand gestures/body movements | *dishonest, deceitful, nervous, lack of self-confidence* |
| Rocking movements | *nervous, lack of self-confidence* |
| Pacing back and forth | *nervous, lack of self-confidence, cornered, angry, upset* |
| Frequent hand-to-face contact/ resting your head in your hands | *dishonest, deceitful, nervous, tired, bored* |
| Hidden hands | *deceptive, guilty, insincere* |
| Speaking from behind barriers (podiums, lecterns, tables) | *dishonest, deceitful, formality, withdrawn, distancing oneself, unconcerned, not interested, superior* |
| Speaking from an elevated position | *superiority, dominant, judgemental* |
| Speaking indoors behind a desk | *bureaucratic, uncaring, removed, distant, uninvolved* |
| Touching and/or rubbing nose | *doubt, disagreement, nervous, deceitful* |
| Touching and/or rubbing eyes | *doubt, disagreement, nervous, deceitful* |
| Pencil chewing/hand pinching | *lack of self-confidence, doubt* |
| Jingling money in pockets | *nervous, lack of self-confidence, lack of self-control, deceitful (hint: empty change from your pockets beforehand)* |
| Constant throat clearing | *nervous, lack of self-confidence* |
| Drumming on table, tapping feet, twitching, etc. | *nervous, hostile, anxious, impatient, bored* |
| Head in hand | *bored, tired, frustrated* |

## NEGATIVELY PERCEIVED NON-VERBAL COMMUNICATION – CONTINUED –

| Clenched hands | anger, hostile, uncooperative |
|---|---|
| Locked ankles/squeezed hands | deceitful, apprehensive, nervous, tense, aggressive |
| Palm to back of neck | frustration, anger, irritation, hostility |
| Tight-lipped | nervous, deceitful, angry, hostile |
| Licking lips | nervous, deceitful |
| Frequent blinking | nervous, deceitful, inattentive |
| Slumping posture | nervousness, poor self-control |
| Raising voice/high-pitched tone of voice | nervous, hostile, deceitful |
| Shrugging shoulders | unconcerned, indifferent |

## BOX 3.6: POSITIVELY PERCEIVED NON-VERBAL COMMUNICATION

| Excellent eye contact | honest, open, competent, caring, empathetic sincere, dedicated, confident, knowledgeable, interested |
|---|---|
| Sitting slightly forward in chair | interested, enthusiastic, concerned, cooperative |
| Open hands | open, sincere |
| Speaking outdoors in low-wind conditions | dedicated, hardworking, involved, concerned |
| Hand to chest/heart region | open, honest, dedicated, sincere |
| Erect posture | self-confident, self-controlled, assertive, determined |
| Lowering voice | self-assured, honest, caring |

# STEP 4
## Prepare messages

**4.1:** *Prepare* lists of stakeholders and their concerns

**4.2:** *Prepare* clear and concise messages

**4.3:** *Prepare* targeted messages

# STEP 4
## Prepare messages

**4.1:** *Prepare* lists of stakeholders and their concerns

**4.2:** *Prepare* clear and concise messages

**4.3:** *Prepare* targeted messages

# 4.1: PREPARE LISTS OF STAKEHOLDERS AND THEIR CONCERNS

## I. Stakeholders

Every emergency typically involves a different set of stakeholders including the public and other interested, affected or influential parties (**BOX 4.1**). Stakeholders can be distinguished by their potential to affect outcomes, their credibility with other stakeholders, and their current relationship with the public health agency (for example, apathetic, neutral. supportive, non-supportive, critical, adversarial, or ambivalent). Each stakeholder will also have a distinctive set of questions and concerns that may be voiced by the media.

## II. Stakeholder concerns

One important step in preparing target messages is identifying, understanding and addressing the questions and concerns of important stakeholders (**BOX 4.2**). Messages can then be developed and delivered in response to these. Such questions and concerns typically fall into three categories:

- **Overarching** – for example, "What do people most need to know about the event"?
- **Informational** – for example, "How many staff do you have"?
- **Challenging** – for example, "Why should we trust what you are telling us"? "How many people have to die before you take more aggressive action"? "Can you guarantee that people are safe"? "What are you not telling us"?

Although lists of specific stakeholder questions and concerns are typically generated by members of the communication team, they can also be generated through empirical research, including:

- media content analysis (print, radio and television);
- analysis of web site material;
- document review, including public meeting records, public hearing records and legislative transcripts;
- reviews of complaint logs, hotline logs, toll-free number logs and media logs;
- focused interviews with subject-matter experts;
- facilitated workshops or discussion sessions with individuals very familiar with the issues;
- focus groups; and
- surveys.

These techniques are an important means of listening to stakeholder concerns and obtaining feedback, and have been applied to a wide variety of public health issues. **ANNEX 6** contains a list of questions frequently asked by journalists and the public during natural or intentional outbreaks of disease. Recent empirical research indicates that a large percentage of the questions and concerns raised by stakeholders in emergency situations can be identified in advance using the above techniques.

**BOX 4.1: EXAMPLES OF STAKEHOLDERS DURING A MAJOR DISEASE OUTBREAK**

- governmental and nongovernmental authorities;
- the media;
- public at large and at risk;
- victims and their families;
- emergency response personnel;
- public health authorities and agencies (local, regional, provincial, national and international);
- physicians, nurses, paramedics and other healthcare personnel;
- veterinarians;
- fire department personnel;
- police and other law enforcement personnel;
- hospital personnel;
- health agency employees;
- families of emergency responders, law enforcement personnel, hospital personnel, and health agency employees;
- government agencies (regulatory and non-regulatory) at all levels;
- employees of other responding organizations;
- politicians/legislators/elected officials;
- union officials and labour advocates;
- legal professionals;
- contractors;
- consultants;
- suppliers/vendors;
- ethnic populations;
- racial populations;
- minority populations;
- institutionalized populations;
- elderly populations;
- religious groups;
- special language groups;
- disabled populations;
- homeless people;
- home-bound populations;
- other vulnerable populations;
- illiterate populations;
- tourists or business travellers and their relatives;
- local residents that are out of town and their relatives;
- security personnel;
- service and maintenance personnel;
- advisory panels;
- nongovernmental organizations (NGOs);
- educational leaders and community (all levels);
- scientific leaders and community;
- business leaders and community;
- military leaders; and
- professional societies.

### BOX 4.2: POTENTIAL CONCERNS IN A PUBLIC HEALTH EMERGENCY

- informational concerns – who, what, where, when, why and how?
- human health concerns
  - one's own
  - children
  - parents
  - friends and family
  - elderly persons
  - expectant mothers
  - special populations
  - others;
- pet concerns;
- livestock concerns;
- wildlife concerns;
- safety concerns;
- ecological and environmental concerns;
- economic concerns;
- quality-of-life concerns;
- equity and fairness concerns;
- cultural and symbolic concerns;
- legal and regulatory concerns;
- honesty and openness concerns;
- transparency and access-to-information concerns;
- accountability concerns;
- future-generational concerns;
- ethical and morality concerns;
- change concerns;
- chaos and loss-of-control concerns;
- panic concerns; and
- trust concerns.

## III. Preparing a matrix of stakeholder concerns

Once the lists of stakeholders and their concerns during a specific emergency situation are produced, a very useful next step can be to develop a "matrix" showing the stakeholders on one axis and their questions and concerns on the other (**FIGURE THREE**). Once complete, such a matrix can be supplemented by additional information entered into the boxes. For example, individual stakeholder concerns can be classified as:

(1) high concern;
(2) medium concern;
(3) low concern; or
(4) not applicable.

One advantage of the resulting matrix is that it can then be used as a resource-allocation guide. Boxes with the highest number of entries (or with the highest number of "high-concern" designations) would be prioritized and addressed first.

STEP 4: Prepare messages

## FIGURE THREE: MATRIX OF STAKEHOLDERS AND THEIR CONCERNS

| Stakeholders | Concerns | | | | | | | | | | | | | |
|---|---|---|---|---|---|---|---|---|---|---|---|---|---|---|
| | Human health | Trust | Safety | Environmental | Information | Ethics | Economics | Responsibility | Legal | Process | Pets/livestock | Religious | Fairness | Other |
| Governmental and nongovernmental authorities | | | | | | | | | | | | | | |
| Public at large and at risk | | | | | | | | | | | | | | |
| Media | | | | | | | | | | | | | | |
| Victims and their families | | | | | | | | | | | | | | |
| Emergency response personnel | | | | | | | | | | | | | | |
| Public health personnel | | | | | | | | | | | | | | |
| Physicians/nurses/ veterinarians | | | | | | | | | | | | | | |
| Law enforcement personnel | | | | | | | | | | | | | | |
| Hospital personnel | | | | | | | | | | | | | | |
| Health agency employees | | | | | | | | | | | | | | |
| Other | | | | | | | | | | | | | | |

# 4.2: PREPARE CLEAR AND CONCISE MESSAGES

A key step in effective media communication is to develop clear and concise messages that address stakeholder questions and concerns. In addition to generating a large number of such questions and concerns, emergency situations are also likely to generate strong feelings of anxiety, anger, frustration, fear and outrage. Messages that address stakeholder concerns should therefore be based on what the target audience most needs to know or most wants to know.

Clear and concise messages can be developed through brainstorming sessions with a message-development team typically consisting of a subject-matter expert, a communication specialist, a policy/legal/management expert, and a facilitator. Such sessions typically produce a set of talking points and key messages. The sessions can also be used to produce keywords as a memory aid for the talking points. Keywords are typically more easily accessed and recalled by spokespersons than narratives and scripts. Most people have difficulty memorizing or delivering scripts but can deliver agreed-upon key words using their own words to form whole sentences.

Talking points, key messages, key words and background materials can all be contained in a media-briefing book (see below). Ideally, this book should be produced in advance for all major emergency scenarios. The most important message in the briefing book will be the overarching message containing the information that an organization most wants people to know in relation to a specific issue or topic. This message can also be put into the opening statement at a presentation, media interview or news conference relating to the issue or topic.

## I. Preparing message maps

One of the most powerful tools for preparing clear and concise messages is the "message map" (**FIGURE FOUR**). A message map consists of detailed and hierarchically organized information that can be used to respond to anticipated questions or concerns. It is a visual aid that provides at a glance the organization's messages on high-concern issues. The message map template enables spokespersons to meet the demands of the public, the media and other interested parties for timely, accurate, clear, concise, consistent, credible and relevant information. The message map can also serve as "a port in a storm" when questioning by journalists or others becomes intense or aggressive. Message maps also allow organizations to develop messages in advance of emergencies and once developed, their effectiveness can be tested through focus groups and other empirical studies.

**STEP 4: Prepare messages**

### FIGURE FOUR: MESSAGE MAP TEMPLATE

Stakeholder:
Question or Concern:

| Key Message 1 | Key Message 2 | Key Message 3 |
|---|---|---|
|  |  |  |
| Supporting Information 1-1 | Supporting Information 2-1 | Supporting Information 3-1 |
|  |  |  |
| Supporting Information 1-2 | Supporting Information 2-2 | Supporting Information 3-2 |
|  |  |  |
| Supporting Information 1-3 | Supporting Information 2-3 | Supporting Information 3-3 |
|  |  |  |

The top section of the message map identifies the stakeholder or audience for whom the messages are intended as well as the specific question or concern being addressed. The next layer of the message map contains the 3 key messages which can function individually or collectively as a response to a stakeholder question or concern. These key messages are intended to address the information needs of a wide variety of audiences.

The three key messages can also serve individually or collectively as a media sound bite – the quote in a media story attributed to a spokesperson. Sound bites are an essential element in effective media communication as short, quotable messages will often be played repeatedly by the media. They often will also be quoted by other sources of information. Speaking in sound bites helps to ensure that prepared key messages are carried in news stories. Reporters and editors almost always cut interview material into sound bites.

The final section of the message map contains supporting information arranged in blocks of 3 under each key message. This supporting information amplifies the key messages by providing additional facts or details. Supporting information can also take the form of visuals, analogies, personal stories or citations of credible information sources.

As a strategic tool, a message map provides multiple benefits. It provides a handy reference for leaders and spokespersons who must respond swiftly to questions on topics where timeliness and accuracy are crucial. Multiple spokespersons can work from the same message map to ensure the rapid dissemination of consistent and core messages across a wide spectrum of communication outlets. Message maps provide a unifying framework for disseminating information on a wide range of public health issues. Message maps also minimize the chance of "speaker's regret" at saying something inappropriate or not saying something that should have been said. A printed copy of the message map allows spokespersons during interviews to "check off" the talking points they want to make in order of their importance. This helps to prevent omissions of key facts or mis-statements that could provoke misunderstandings, controversy or outrage.

Message maps were developed as a specialized tool for communicating effectively in high-stress, high-concern or emotionally charged situations. Numerous public health agencies have conducted message-mapping projects focused on a range of public health issues, including bio-terrorist events and disease outbreaks. Emergency events that have already been mapped include smallpox (**FIGURE FIVE**), plague, botulism, viral haemorrhagic fevers, tularemia and pandemic flu.

One important lesson learned from message-mapping exercises is that the process of generating message maps can be as important as the end product. Message-mapping exercises involve teams of scientists, communication specialists and individuals with policy expertise, and often reveal a diversity of viewpoints on the same question, issue or concern. Gaps in message maps often provide early warning that a message is incomplete providing scientists and issue-management teams with an opportunity to focus their efforts on filling the information gaps. Message-mapping exercises also frequently identify changes needed in organizational strategies and policies.

The crucial final step in message-map construction is to conduct systematic message testing using standardized procedures. Message testing should begin by asking subject-matter experts not directly involved in the original message-mapping process to validate the accuracy of the information given. Message testing should then be conducted with individuals or groups who have the characteristics to serve as surrogates for key internal and external target audiences. Finally, sharing and testing messages with partner organizations will promote message consistency and coordination. Once developed, message maps can be brought together to produce the media briefing book referred to above. They can also be used individually or collectively for use in news conferences, media interviews, information forums and exchanges, public meetings, web sites, telephone hotline scripts and fact sheets or brochures.

### FIGURE FIVE: SAMPLE SMALLPOX MESSAGE MAP – WITH KEYWORDS IN ITALICS

Stakeholder: Public

Question or Concern: How contagious is smallpox?

| Key Message 1 | Key Message 2 | Key Message 3 |
|---|---|---|
| Smallpox *spreads slowly* compared to many other diseases. | This allows *time to trace* those who have come into contact with the disease. | Those who have been traced *can be vaccinated* to prevent illness. |
| **Supporting Information 1-1** | **Supporting Information 2-1** | **Supporting Information 3-1** |
| People are only infectious when the rash appears. | The incubation period for the disease is 10–14 days | People who have never been vaccinated are the most important to vaccinate. |
| **Supporting Information 1-2** | **Supporting Information t 2-2** | **Supporting Information 3-2** |
| Smallpox typically requires hours of face-to-face contact. | Resources are available for tracing contacts. | Adults who were vaccinated as children may still have some immunity. |
| **Supporting Information 1-3** | **Supporting Information 2-3** | **Supporting Information 3-3** |
| There are no carriers without symptoms. | Finding people who have been exposed and vaccinating them has proved successful in the past. | Adequate vaccine is on hand. |

> **INFORMATION POINT: Examples of technical terms used in public health that may not be understood by the public**
>
> - Age-adjusted mortality rate
> - Attributable risk
> - Carcinogen
> - Confidence interval
> - Control group
> - Dose-response
> - Epidemiology
> - Incidence rate
> - Morbidity
> - Mortality
> - Mutagen
> - Odds ratio
> - Prevalence
> - Prophylactic
> - Reference dose
> - Relative risk
> - Standard deviation
> - Statistical significance
> - Surveillance
> - Toxicology
> - Variance
> - Vector

## II. Preparing and distributing a news release

If at all possible, information to be included in a news release should be prepared in advance. During an actual emergency situation, the time pressure is likely to immense. As a result, what has been prepared beforehand will be crucial. If news release templates for the major categories of public health emergencies most likely to occur have already been prepared this will help to get the process off to a good start.

### 1. What is a news release?

A news release[1] tells reporters the basic who, what, when, where, why and how of an event. Most importantly, a news release should quickly convey the vital information. Reporters use news releases to help determine whether they will cover a story, and to gather the information needed to write it. Because reporters often receive many news releases, it is normally important to grab their attention and convince them of the story's value. During an emergency this will be less relevant as reporters will already be on board. In all cases, the news release must meet their deadlines.

### 2. How are news releases prepared?

News releases generally follow a standard format designed to quickly give the reporter all the information they need. The "inverted pyramid" style of writing should be followed in which the most important and essential information appears first followed by supporting information. Sometimes this is referred to as "bottom line up front" (BLUF) because reporters are often extremely busy and may not have time to read the entire release.

In addition to answering or addressing the basic questions, the release should also express concern, provide guidance (if appropriate), and give details about how further information will be disseminated. If possible, the release should also give telephone numbers or contacts for more information or assistance. If possible and appropriate, the release should include direct quotes from the agency leader.

The more that news releases are written like news articles, the greater the chance the media will use them (or selected paragraphs) in their entirety. This will increase the probability that the agency's messages will be accurately reported and repeated. If a release cannot be issued, consideration should be given to providing the media with a fact sheet or list of frequently asked questions (FAQs). In this way, factual information can at least be put in the hands of the media, greatly reducing the risk of misunderstandings. As with all communication materials, news releases need to be approved using the agency's clearance and approval protocol (for example, by a subject-matter expert, the agency director, or the public information officer).

---

1 The term "news release" and "press release" are often used synonymously. The term "press release" harks back to an earlier time when newspapers dominated.

## 3. Essential elements of a news release

**FIGURE SIX** shows a sample template for a news release. Although it can be used as shown, the sample is meant only to provide guidance as a single template structure will not work for every situation and should be modified for local application. The first paragraph is designed to capture the interest of the reporter and should contain the most important information of the release remembering to:

- keep it very short;
- limit paragraph to 1–3 sentences at most;
- use plain language; and
- avoid using acronyms and jargon.

The length of the entire news release must in fact be kept short (1–2 pages double-spaced). Quotations should be used whenever possible to add a "human side" to the story, and should:

- support statements made in the first lead paragraph;
- be from a significant person;
- add information; and
- be included within the first three or four paragraphs.

> **INFORMATION POINT: Contents of a news release**
> - Insert headline.
> - Insert the key messages to the public.
> - Insert 2–3 sentences describing the current situation.
> - Insert quote from the lead spokesperson or agency head demonstrating leadership and concern.
> - List actions currently being taken.
> - List actions that will be taken next.
> - List information on possible reactions of the public and on ways the public can help.
> - List contact information, ways to get more information from the agency, links to other organizations and other resources.

## 4. Coordinating news releases with internal and external partners

- identify (and if appropriate) consult with partner organizations interested in, or affected by, the news release;
- ensure all partners receive a copy of the release before it is provided to the media;
- identify procedures for sharing the news release with internal staff;
- determine how information will be released and who will do the releasing;
- prepare and distribute joint news releases; and
- assist partners in developing their own news release.

STEP 4: Prepare messages

## FIGURE SIX: SAMPLE NEWS RELEASE TEMPLATE

[ORGANIZATION'S NAME ON LETTERHEAD]

NEWS RELEASE

FOR IMMEDIATE RELEASE

For more information, contact:

[DATE]

[Name of internal media representative/contact person]

[Name of organization]

[Telephone number]

[Fax number]

[Email address]

[After-hours telephone number]

[Web site for more information]

[Headline goes here, initial cap, bold]

[CITY, State] – [Date] – [Text goes here, double-spaced, indented paragraphs]

[First paragraph: short (less than 30–35 words); contains the most important information]

[Second paragraph: contains the who, what, why, where, when of the story. Try to include a quote from the lead spokesperson or agency leadership within the first few paragraphs]

*If the news release is more than one page long, use:*

– more –

*Centre the word at the bottom of the page, then continue onto the next page with a brief description of the headline, and page number as follows:*

[Shortened headline] – Page 2

[The last paragraph should be an organization boilerplate, which is a brief description of the organization, and any information considered useful for people to know, such as type of organization, its location and web site address]

*At the end of the release put:*

End or ###

*centred at the bottom. This lets the reporter/reader know they have come to the end.*

End

## III. Preparing messages for media interviews

Messages for potential media interviews during emergencies can be prepared using the five-step model presented in **BOX 4.3**.

**BOX 4.3: A FIVE-STEP MODEL FOR PREPARING MESSAGES FOR POTENTIAL MEDIA INTERVIEWS DURING AN EMERGENCY**

| Answers should: | By: |
|---|---|
| 1. Express empathy, listening, caring or compassion as a first statement. | • using personal pronouns, such as "I" "we" "our" or "us";<br>• indicating through actions, body language and words that you share the concerns of those affected by events;<br>• acknowledging the legitimacy of fear and emotion;<br>• using a personal story, if appropriate (for example, "My family…"; and<br>• bridging to the key messages. |
| 2. State the key messages. | • limiting the total number of words to no more than 27;<br>• limiting the total length to no more than 9 seconds;<br>• using positive, constructive and solution-oriented words as appropriate; and<br>• setting messages apart with introductory words, pauses and inflections. |
| 3. State supporting information. | • using three additional facts;<br>• using well thought out and tested visual material, including graphics, maps, pictures, video clips, animation, photographs and analogies;<br>• using a personal story; and<br>• citing credible third parties or other credible sources of information. |
| 4. Repeat the key messages. | • summarizing or emphasizing the key messages. |
| 5. State future actions. | • listing specific next steps; and<br>• providing contact information for obtaining additional information, if appropriate. |

## IV. Principles of message preparation

The preparation of all the above types of message should be guided by the theories and principles of effective media communication. For example, "mental noise theory" is one of the main constructs in the emergency communication literature. This theory recognizes that when people are upset they often have difficulty comprehending or remembering information. This effect can reduce a person's ability to process information by more than 80%, and the challenge for risk communicators, is therefore to:

- overcome the barriers that mental noise creates;
- produce accurate messages for diverse audiences in diverse social and cultural contexts; and
- achieve maximum communication effectiveness within the constraints posed by mental noise.

Professional communicators use a variety of means to overcome interference in message reception. For example, they limit the number of key messages to a maximum of three using no more than 9 seconds or 27 words to express the necessary information. They construct messages that are clearly understandable by the target audience – message maps produced by public health agencies in developed nations are typically constructed to be easily understood by an adult with a 6th to 8th grade education. This can be tested using the "readability" utility contained in a number of word-processing programmes.

Additional solutions include:

- Adhering to the "primacy/recency" or "first/last" principle. This principle states that the most important messages should occupy the first and last position in a list. In high-stress situations listeners tend to focus most on (and remember) information that they hear first and last. Messages that are in the middle of a list are often not heard. Focus-group testing confirms that people often cannot recall middle-placed messages.
- Citing third parties or sources that would be perceived as credible by the receiving audience. The greater the extent to which messages are supported and corroborated by credible third party sources, the greater the level of trust and the less likely it is that mental noise will interfere with the ability to comprehend messages.
- Providing a preamble to the message map that indicates genuine empathy, listening, caring and compassion – crucial factors in establishing trust in high-concern, high-stress situations. The greater the extent to which individuals and organizations are perceived to be empathetic, caring, listening and compassionate, the less likely it is that mental noise will interfere with message comprehension.
- Using graphics, visual aids, analogies and narratives (such as personal stories) can increase an individual's ability to hear, understand and recall a message by more than 50%.
- Constructing messages while recognizing the dominant role of negative thinking in high-concern situations. According to negative dominance theory (asymmetry theory), people tend to focus more on the negative than on the positive in emotionally charged situations, with resulting high levels of anxiety and exaggerated fears. Potential solutions include:
  - avoiding unnecessary, indefensible or non-productive uses of absolutes, and of the words "no", "not", "never", "nothing" and "none";
  - balancing or countering a negative key message with positive, constructive or solution-oriented key messages; and
  - providing three or more positive points to counter a single negative point or bad news. It is important to note in this regard that a trust-building message is a positive response in and of itself and can count as one or more of the positives. It is also important to recognize that health agencies have very limited control over what messages the media will emphasize. The media control which messages will be cited, what visibility they will be given, and how often they will be repeated. As a result, many positive messages may fall by the wayside. This is especially likely to be the case if the positives are hypothetical or predictive and the negatives are matters of fact.
- Presenting the full message map using the repetitive structure found in the "Tell me, Tell me more, Tell me again model" (the "Triple T Model") namely:
  - *Tell* people the information in summary form (i.e., the three key messages;
  - *Tell them more* (i.e., the supporting information); and
  - *Tell people again* what was told in summary form (i.e., repeat the three key messages). The greater the extent to which messages are repeated and heard through various channels, the less likely it is that mental noise will interfere with the ability to comprehend them.
- Developing key messages and supporting information that address important risk perception, outrage and fear factors such as trust, benefits, control, voluntariness, dread, fairness, reversibility, catastrophic potential, effects on children, morality, origin and familiarity. The risk-perception, outrage and fear factors listed in **BOX 4.4** are among those causing the highest levels of worry, anxiety and mental noise. Research indicates that the greater the extent to which these factors are addressed in messaging, the less likely it is that mental noise will interfere with the ability to comprehend messages.

# STEP 4: Prepare messages

> **BOX 4.4: RISK-PERCEPTION AND FEAR FACTORS**
>
> **Risks and threats are generally more worrisome, anxiety producing, stressful and fearsome if they are perceived to:**
>
> - be caused by an invisible or non-observed agent;
> - be involuntary or imposed;
> - be inequitably distributed;
> - be inescapable;
> - be under the control of others, especially those we don't trust;
> - arise from an unfamiliar or novel sources;
> - result from man-made rather than natural sources;
> - cause hidden and irreversible damage;
> - pose some particular danger to small children, pregnant women or more generally to future generations;
> - threaten a form of death (or illness/injury) that is particularly dreaded;
> - threaten or harm identifiable rather than anonymous or theoretical victims;
> - pose a personal threat by singling you out from others;
> - offer little or no compensating benefits;
> - be new and poorly understood by science; and
> - be subject to contradictory statements.

Recent studies also indicate that it is vital that key messages be concisely stated if they are offered to the news media as sound bites or quotes. For example, an analysis of 10 years of print and media coverage of emergencies in the United States found:

- the average length of a sound bite in the print media was 27 words;
- the average duration of a sound bite in the broadcast media was nine seconds;
- the average number of messages reported in both the print and broadcast media was three; and
- quotes most likely to be used as sound bites contained compassion, conviction and optimism.

Adherence to the 27-word/9-second/3-message limitations (the "27/9/3" template) will help to ensure that spokespersons are quoted accurately and completely in interviews and elsewhere in the media. Sound bites are typically supplemented with supporting facts, information or proofs. The same principles that guide message construction guide the development of supporting information. Proof points, especially when they are highly complex or technical, are often held in reserve to support a particular message if challenged.

> **INFORMATION POINT: Guidelines for preparing clear and concise messages during public health emergencies**
>
> - identify what you most want the target audience to know;
> - identify what you need to do to correct misperceptions or erroneous information;
> - prepare three key messages that communicate your overarching (core) talking points;
> - prepare supporting message points for each key message;
> - develop supporting material for each message (for example, visuals, examples, quotes, personal stories, analogies, endorsements by credible third parties, or directions for obtaining additional information);
> - keep messages simple and short;
> - document in writing the recommended messages and supporting material; and
> - practise delivery.

# 4.3: PREPARE TARGETED MESSAGES

People experiencing extreme high stress and anxiety are a key audience. Reaching these individuals through the media requires in-depth awareness and understanding of their feelings and state of mind. Communicating badly can lead to additional stress, anxiety, confusion and resentment. Communicate well and people are more likely to understand, accept, cope and adjust.

## I. Extreme stress and anxiety

It is common for individuals involved in a public health emergency – including victims and emergency responders – to experience extreme stress and anxiety, and to exhibit a wide arrange of thoughts, feelings and behaviours. Extreme stress and anxiety can overwhelm an individual's ability to cope.

The most common reactions to extreme stress and anxiety that impair the way information is received during or after a public health emergency include:

| Reaction | Identifying characteristics |
| --- | --- |
| **Cognitive** | Confusion, poor problem-solving ability, lowered alertness, poor judgement, difficulty calculating, heightened anxiety, impaired memory, easily distracted, inattention to detail, neglect of personal hygiene, neglect of responsibilities, disorientation and hopelessness. |
| **Physical** | Rapid heart beat, tremors, intestinal upset, nausea, sleep disturbance, elevated blood pressure, chills, dizziness, chest pains, headaches and fatigue. |
| **Behavioural** | Difficulty sleeping, appetite change, easily startled, uncontrollable crying, isolation from others, fatigue, nightmares, hyper-vigilance, withdrawal, avoidance, substance abuse (such as increased alcohol and tobacco use), eating disorders and sexual dysfunction. |
| **Emotional** | Guilt, fear, shock, sadness, irritability, anger, disbelief, emotional numbness, panic attacks and depressed mood. |

In addition to these reactions, research based on interviews with individuals experiencing grief indicates that such individuals may go through the following processes: trauma, shock, denial (by ignoring warnings or ignoring messages to take protective actions), anger (for example, in the form of emotional outbursts or assigning blame to others), bargaining (trying to find something to mitigate or solve the problem), depression, acceptance of loss and forgiveness.

One highly stressed group often overlooked as a target audience for emergency communication is first responders, health care workers and their families. For example, their stress levels are likely to be significantly higher if they are not in receipt of timely and accurate information on the status and protection of their own family members. Failure to provide such information can lead to absenteeism or negatively impact upon performance of critical job responsibilities.

Recent trauma survivors may also have difficulties in concentrating, and may tend to avoid any reminders of anything associated with the trauma. As a result:

- communications need to be simple;
- communications need to be repeated; and
- checks need to be conducted to ensure that key messages have been understood.

## INFORMATION POINT: Summary guidelines for simplifying interviews, presentations and messages

**Meet the audience more than halfway**

- the higher the level of stress, fear or anxiety, the greater the need to simplify the language and to carefully structure communications;
- use the readability utility included with most word-processing software to measure the readability level of the information; and
- aim to produce messages that are easily understood by the target audience.

**Use clear language**

- provide no more than 3 message points or ideas at a time;
- use simple and correct grammar;
- use short sentences;
- be careful when providing numbers – these can easily be misinterpreted or misunderstood; and
- avoid the use of jargon, acronyms and new terms, and:
  - define new terms so that the target audience can understand them
  - use short sentences to define new terms
  - provide a glossary
  - introduce the concept before introducing a new term or explain the new term soon after using it
  - if possible, ask the audience to identify terms that are not understood
  - check frequently for understanding
  - use new terms only if it is important for the target audience to know and remember them
  - be careful when using technical words that have a different meaning from their common usage.

**Delivery**

- test messages with people who have only a limited knowledge of the topic;
- provide your audience with advance warning when complex or difficult material will be shared;
- break down complex topics into smaller parts;
- use the "Triple T Model" for presenting complex information – tell your audience briefly what you are going to tell them; tell them more about each point; tell them again briefly what you told them;
- ask questions designed to uncover the intuitive mental models used by the audience to understand the topic – correct misconceptions if needed;
- develop materials with which people can interact, such as material on web sites;
- use the active voice for writing and speaking; and
- provide complex information in tiers or layers of information that increase gradually in complexity.

**Presentation**

- use visuals (for example, graphics, drawings, maps, charts, flowcharts, paintings, photographs, video and highlighted text) to enhance comprehension;
- use simple graphics
  - whose main point can be grasped in less than 3 seconds
  - that contain no more than 1–2 main points
  - that put the main point of the graphic in writing in the graphic itself
  - that use one graphic per point in a sequenced set of graphics
  - that use simple formats, such as bar graphs and pie charts;
- use flowcharts or outlines for complicated issues;
- use colour;
- use colours to enhance meaning, but do not depend on colours to convey your message;
- beware of colours that are difficult to distinguish from surrounding colours;
- when using black and white, it is often difficult to distinguish various shades of grey;
- beware of colours that convey their own messages, which can vary between cultures;
- determine if the material is consistent with culturally accepted ways of presenting or accessing information; and
- respect and allow for the diverse nature of the target audience – for example, enlarge the type face and font size for audiences who are elderly or sight-impaired.

STEP 4: Prepare messages

> **INFORMATION POINT: Communicating effectively to individuals experiencing extreme stress or anxiety**
>
> **Recognize that communications success depends upon:**
> - a trusting relationship between communicator and audience;
> - the attitude and knowledge of the communicator; and
> - the clarity and salience of the message.
>
> **Tailor messages to specific groups, such as:**
> - first responders;
> - health-care workers;
> - victims;
> - families of victims; and
> - parents.
>
> **Consider messages that:**
> - create a feeling of competence ("Help people to help themselves");
> - encourage people to create support systems to supplement formal and external assistance; and
> - channel negative responses into positive action.

## STEP 5
### Identify media outlets and media activities

**5.1:** *Identify* available media outlets
**5.2:** *Identify* the most effective media outlets
**5.3:** *Identify* media activities for the first 24–72 hours

# STEP 5
## Identify media outlets and media activities

**5.1:** *Identify* available media outlets
**5.2:** *Identify* the most effective media outlets
**5.3:** *Identify* media activities for the first 24–72 hours

# 5.1: IDENTIFY AVAILABLE MEDIA OUTLETS

In most parts of the world, there is a wide range of potential media and media outlets that can be used to reach the intended or targeted audience. The choice of media and the strategies to be used may need to be reviewed as the emergency develops because people may change their listening, reading and other information-seeking habits. Any of the following communication outlets can be used on a broad or much smaller targeted scale.

## I. Potential media communication outlets

- news releases;
- news briefings and conferences (in person and by telephone);
- interviews on television or radio news programmes;
- interviews on radio or television talk shows;
- call-in programmes (radio or television);
- interviews in weekly or monthly journals and magazines;
- interviews in trade or professional publications;
- briefings for editorial boards of news organizations;
- web sites – including the agency's public site as well as dedicated sites for specific users or events;
- public address systems;
- public service announcements;
- telephone hotlines and toll-free numbers;
- email;
- faxes;
- short wave radio;
- paid advertisements;
- flyers, brochures and circulars;
- presentations for local community organizations, service clubs, religious organizations and voluntary organizations;
- participation in already-planned community events;
- billboards;
- direct mailings;
- displays and exhibits;
- CDs;
- audio tapes;
- information centres;
- text messages on mobile telephones;
- mobile and cell phone voice mail;
- pagers;
- newsletters; and
- folk and traditional media (for example, storytelling).

Although the mass media can be used to reach large numbers of people quickly, a number of the smaller media outlets listed above may provide a better way of reaching some populations. These include those that do not routinely use mass media channels or who do not have confidence in mainstream media or official government pronouncements. In these situations, lower technology options (such as traditional and folk channels, and particularly person-to-person communication networks) may be the more appropriate outreach mechanism. Factors that limit the usefulness of print and broadcast mass media outlets in emergencies include:

## STEP 5: Identify media outlets and media activities

- print and broadcast mass media may not be the dominant way people receive information;
- people have an expanding number of technologies that can used for communication;
- people typically seek out and receive information from multiple sources; and
- mass media communication systems are often highly vulnerable to technical failure due to their complex infrastructures.

Another serious limitation of many mass media and other approaches is that they are strictly one-way communication vehicles. Although they can be an efficient means of disseminating information, they lack the capacity to provide meaningful feedback and dialogue. Typically such channels:

- are not interactive or two-way;
- do not allow or encourage the public to become a true partner in decision-making;
- can not provide feedback on how messages are being received; and
- do not give the public a real voice, except as interpreted by the media themselves.

By contrast, the following media outlets can offer opportunities to obtain meaningful feedback as part of a two-way dialogue with stakeholders, especially when carefully planned and organized:

- advisory committees and forums;
- panels;
- expert availability sessions;
- workshops;
- public discussion forums;
- open houses;
- public meetings;
- public hearings;
- information exchanges;
- internet chat rooms, interactive web sites and news media web sites that invite feedback;
- text and SMS messaging using mobile and cell phones; and
- consultations.

Many of these potential feedback mechanisms may not however be practical in an emergency, and as a result, many will most frequently be used before or after an event (for example, as part of follow-up and evaluation). For all these reasons, engagement with the mass news media should always be only one aspect of a larger communication strategy during public health emergencies. To facilitate this, the worksheet presented in **FIGURE SEVEN** should be used in advance to identify and profile media outlets serving the community and a media-communications strategy planned accordingly. During the planning process each media outlet's past coverage should be considered. It should be remembered that during an emergency many different media outlets will be seeking out individuals for news and thus only so much can be planned.

**STEP 5: Identify media outlets and media activities**

## FIGURE SEVEN: IDENTIFYING AND PROFILING MEDIA OUTLETS

| Media | Contact information | Position and past coverage of the issue |
|---|---|---|
| Newspapers | | |
| | | |
| | | |
| | | |
| Radio stations | | |
| | | |
| | | |
| | | |
| Television stations | | |
| | | |
| | | |
| | | |
| Newsletters | | |
| | | |
| | | |
| | | |
| Bulletin boards (conventional and computerized) | | |
| | | |
| | | |
| | | |
| Web sites | | |
| | | |
| | | |
| | | |
| Community newsletters | | |
| | | |
| | | |
| | | |
| Traditional and folk media | | |
| | | |
| | | |
| | | |
| Other | | |
| | | |
| | | |
| | | |

**This form should be adapted to meet local needs**

# 5.2: IDENTIFY THE MOST EFFECTIVE MEDIA OUTLETS

Each of the potential media outlets listed above will have their own advantages and disadvantages. During an emergency situation, successful media communication will depend upon a number of factors, including the use of the most appropriate and effective methods of transmitting the prepared messages. Factors to consider in determining the best method for such effective communication include:

- target audience;
- complexity of messages;
- degree of urgency;
- timeliness;
- cost;
- staffing needs;
- media interest; and
- the message itself and how it will be used.

Identifying the media outlets that will be most effective and appropriate in any given situation requires an awareness of the characteristics of each, and of their advantages and disadvantages.

## I. Newspapers

### 1. Advantages of newspapers

- often widely read;
- can cover subjects in detail;
- can handle complex issues;
- can include visual material such as illustrations and graphics to help make the point;
- often have specialist reporters (including health reporters);
- notes can be used during the interview;
- may have a separate online edition that is continually updated;
- the story, if positive, remains in online databases for people to find through an internet search for many years afterward; and
- mistakes and errors can be identified and corrected as soon as the next day.

### 2. Disadvantages of newspapers

- there may delays of 24 hours or more before the public receives news through the print media;
- as with all media, misquoting is possible;
- messages can be heavily edited, possibly leaving only inconsequential comments or comments that are taken out of context;
- the story, if negative, remains in online databases for people to find through an internet search for many years afterward; and
- the story may have an undesirable slant.

## 3. Contact with the newspaper

- be prepared to decline an interview invitation – tell the reporter you are not the right person and why, and if possible refer the reporter to the right person; and
- before the interview begins, ask the reporter (at a minimum):
  - what is the specific topic?
  - what information do they want to cover in the interview?
  - will the interview be on the telephone or face-to-face?
  - when will the story run?
  - are they working to a deadline?

## 4. The newspaper interview

- never say anything that is off the record;
- be prepared to give additional background material that will help the reporter to better write their article;
- allow the interview to be recorded – it can help improve accuracy;
- consider making your own recording to check you have not been misquoted;
- before the interview, prepare key messages and responses to anticipated questions; and
- rehearse offering the key messages and sound bites.

# II. Radio

Nearly every household has a radio or access to one. Portable radios help people even in remote areas get access to the news. This medium is excellent for most communication purposes. In some communication approaches, regular radio programming is interrupted and supplemented by emergency broadcasts covering specific emergency events.

## 1. Advantages of radio

- penetrates even remote areas where print materials are not available;
- allows rapid transmission of up-to-the-minute news;
- can be used to provide information focused on a limited geographical area;
- provides a variety of formats and opportunities to get messages to specific audiences;
- if broadcast is live then messages cannot be edited on the programme itself; and
- allows speaker's personality to be expressed better than in print media.

## 2. Disadvantages of radio

- typically allows for only a short amount of preparation time;
- typically very short (less than one minute) thereby requiring extreme brevity in message delivery;
- as with all media, misquoting is possible;
- if a broadcast is not live, messages can be heavily edited, possibly leaving only inconsequential comments or comments that are taken out of context; and
- if a spokesperson is not briefed well on the subject matter, weaknesses can easily be exposed.

### 3. The radio news interview

- often very brief;
- often the reporter has little time for preparation or editing;
- often broadcast live; and
- keys to success:
  - discuss the specific topics to be covered with the reporter before the interview
  - speak in sound bites that ideally are less than 9 seconds in length and contain fewer than 27 words
  - rehearse the key messages
  - use bridging statements to return frequently to the key messages
  - even if someone has been media-trained, they should consult with a media expert if they think the interview will be difficult.

## III. The radio call-in show

- many call-in shows have a bias or political slant;
- the entire interview process becomes the news product;
- discussion can go anywhere because the host and callers determine the direction;
- the host will typically not allow rules to be imposed on the callers;
- some callers enjoy asking provoking questions or being rude – stay calm and don't respond in the same way; and
- call-in questions are sometimes unclear or vague – when unclear about the question or when asked a broad question such as "why are you doing such a horrible job"? demonstrate listening, state the key messages, affirm the positives of what is being done, and ask if the caller has a specific question.

## IV. Television

When done well, television can be very powerful and effective and have the greatest impact of any media. Television interviews, however, tend to be the most difficult of all media formats, so it is essential to be well practised before going on-camera. At the end of the interview, a spokesperson should not move and should stay silent until the producer confirms that transmission has definitely stopped. An off-hand comment said at the end of the interview, when they think it is all over, can ruin everything.

### 1. Advantages of television

- many people get their news from television;
- a good interview or sound bite can have a powerful effect, and can reach many people;
- it allows immediate and rapid transmission of information;
- if the television broadcast is live, a spokesperson cannot be edited on the programme itself (and therefore the context cannot be changed);
- body language can be used to express listening, caring, empathy and compassion; and
- television encourages the use of visuals, such as graphics, photographs, animation, video clips, maps, props and charts, all of which can increase understanding and make information more memorable.

## 2. Disadvantages of television

- the spokesperson is on view, not just their words;
- it is hard to conceal nervousness – body language may let you down;
- as with all media, misquoting is possible;
- if not a live broadcast, messages can be heavily edited leaving only inconsequential comments or comments taken out of context;
- non-verbal communications become much more important; and
- a very bad interview can undermine efforts and ruin an individual's reputation.

## 3. Visual considerations on television

- body language is just as important as what is said;
- appearance and gestures must be consistent with the verbal messages;
- remember what you have been taught about body language;
- maintain steady eye contact with the interviewer at all times, unless you are in a remote studio, in which case you should look directly at the camera;
- remember and rehearse sound bites and key messages;
- smiling says, "I am confident", except when offered at the wrong time (for example, during discussions of loss of life or hardship);
- dress:
  - dress conservatively
  - avoid loud colours, patterns or stripes
  - avoid wearing articles of clothing with visible commercial logos
  - avoid showy or ostentatious jewellery and jewellery that might create a glare;
  - wear long socks when wearing trousers;
  - avoid pure white shirts or blouses because of glare; and
- discuss with the producer the backdrop for the interview – it becomes part of the message.

# V. The chat show

This media outlet can reach specialized audiences (including decision-makers) but can also be very difficult to do well. The approach is likely to work best if you already know the host and/or have watched earlier shows. In general, it is advisable to arrive early, be prepared and to clarify how the interview will be conducted by asking:

- about content;
- who else will be appearing;
- how long it will last;
- if there will be a debate or discussion with the viewing audience; and
- if it will be live or pre-recorded.

# VI. Web sites

## 1. Advantages of web sites

- highly efficient global distribution;
- allows you to say exactly what you want to say in a written form if it is your own web site;
- can be changed and updated quickly;
- provides assurance that your graphics and other visual material will be used;
- can link to other sites for supporting or supplemental information;
- is available long after the information is originally posted; and
- can be rich in information, with multiple layers of depth.

## 2. Disadvantages of web sites

- can be impersonal;
- difficult to convey feelings, empathy, compassion and concern;
- web users are often in a hurry;
- special populations, low-income audiences and others will often have only limited or no access compared to other forms of media; and
- web pages can be in competition for attention with many others.

## 3. Design tips for web sites

- remember that web users typically scan web pages and do not read them word by word;
- remember that users typically read web pages more slowly than other printed material;
- design the web site to allow users to easily find and go to topics that interest them;
- design web pages to be self-explanatory and independent – users should be able to read the page without the need to visit other web pages;
- design the site keeping in mind the different cultural meanings assigned to symbols, signs, words, colours and imagery;
- design the site to allow feedback from users;
- use simple sentence structures;
- use half the words that would be used in an equivalent paper document;
- highlight key words (for example, by using colour, italics or boldface);
- use bulleted and numbered lists to slow down the reader, encouraging them to focus on important points;
- write in the inverted pyramid (bottom line up front) style;
- use hyperlinks to provide more-detailed information;
- check regularly on what is being said about the topic on other web sites; and
- update the web site frequently.

## 4. Web site graphics

- can reinforce messages;
- can elaborate on messages;
- can highlight messages;
- can substitute for text;
- can be slow to load on a user's computer; and
- can be distracting if not done well.

# VII. Traditional and folk media

A wide variety of traditional and folk media communication channels are available for use before, during and after emergencies. These are particularly useful where there is limited access to (or use of) electronic mass media channels – for example, in highly rural areas. Such channels can either be used on their own or they can be used to supplement information provided through mass media channels.

Traditional and folk media communication channels are typically highly diverse. They include storytelling, puppetry, songs, dancing and poetry recitals, as well as the creative use of traditional arts and crafts.

## 1. Ways of integrating traditional/folk and mass media

- radio dramas;
- radio and television spots;
- musical concerts;
- soap operas;
- poetry recitals; and
- cable television channels dedicated to education.

Such integration serves the dual purpose of entertaining and educating the target audience. As with other forms of communication, many of these traditional and folk media channels may not be practical during an emergency. In most cases, these channels are better used before or after an event (for example, as part of follow-up and evaluation).

Traditional and folk media are also part of a larger system of informal media communication. Informal media communication channels include interpersonal contacts and communication through trusted intermediaries. Interpersonal contacts and trusted intermediaries play a key role in informing people and in persuading people to adopt particular attitudes or behaviours. In addition, informal media communication channels address the needs of those who cannot read, while also addressing local interests and concerns in language and idioms that the audience is most familiar with and understands.

## 2. Visual outlets of folk and traditional communication

- dancing;
- designs on fabrics and clothing;
- carvings;
- paintings;
- drawings;
- signs;
- posters and billboards;
- fairs and festivals; and
- miscellaneous arts and crafts.

## 3. Audio outlets

- singing;
- concerts;
- poetry recitals;
- folk tales;
- gong beating;
- drumming;
- funeral dirges;
- proverbs;
- role play;
- street theatre; and
- dramatic recitals.

# 5.3: IDENTIFY MEDIA ACTIVITIES FOR THE FIRST 24–72 HOURS

## I. Characteristics of the first 24–72 hours of an emergency

- events that exceed the normal capacity of the organization, community or systems to respond;
- the need to engage in extraordinary actions and measures;
- the need to respond swiftly;
- unreliable information;
- information overload;
- high demands for information;
- uncertainty in roles, responsibilities and outcomes;
- absence of control;
- outcomes that are highly uncertain;
- fear;
- perceptions of chaos, panic and disorder;
- breakdown of communications;
- unfamiliarity;
- rapid change;
- accelerated and time-sensitive decision-making and action;
- a large commitment of time by top management;
- a large commitment of time by the entire agency infrastructure;
- major redeployment of organizational resources;
- major disruptions in the normal functioning of organizations or communities;
- threats to the organization's reputation;
- a surge in attention by the media; and
- the potential for extremely negative media coverage.

> **INFORMATION POINT: Causes of public health emergencies**
>
> **Public health emergencies can quickly arise following exposure to:**
> - airborne risk agents;
> - food-borne risk agents;
> - waterborne risk agents;
> - vector-borne risk agents;
> - unknown infectious agents;
> - chemical risk agents;
> - toxic materials;
> - biological risk agents; and
> - radiological materials.
>
> **Emergencies can also arise quickly as a result of:**
> - natural disasters;
> - military activities;
> - terrorist activities;
> - political revolutions;
> - accidents, incidents or explosions at industrial or nuclear facilities that result in injuries, deaths, property damage or economic losses;
> - media investigations that discover wrongdoing;
> - official leaks of sensitive information;
> - breeches of security (deliberate and accidental); and
> - scandals.

## II. Communication challenges

All actions taken within this initial phase of a public health emergency are operationally crucial in that first impressions are lasting impressions. The communication challenges faced by an organization during this time typically include:

- extreme pressure on the organization to provide accurate, timely, early, transparent and relevant information;
- a surge in media attention;
- media "thirst" for different angles on the story;
- media sensationalism;
- information voids which if not filled by official sources are often filled by non-official, misinformed and potentially damaging sources;
- communication systems subjected to severe stress and testing;
- communication breakdowns;
- opposing voices seeking visibility for their points of view;
- bad decisions resulting from poor communications and information; and
- unexpected events.

For these reasons it is essential that public health emergencies are both anticipated and prepared for (**BOX 5.1**). In this way, media activities during the first 24–72 hours can more easily be carried out in accordance with the guidelines set out in **BOX 5.2**.

### BOX 5.1: ANTICIPATING AND PREPARING FOR AN EMERGENCY

**Anticipating**
- The specifics of most emergencies (the who, what, where, when, why, and how) cannot for the most part be anticipated.
- The generalities of an emergency (including many of the questions and concerns that will be raised) can be anticipated – it can be assumed that an emergency will arise at some point.
- The responsibility for determining what can be done before, during and after an emergency must be clearly assigned.
- Cooperation and partnership with others (including governmental and nongovernmental organizations) will expand organizational reach and increase resources.
- An emergency communication plan is essential not optional – it will help in anticipating what might happen and reacting accordingly.

**Preparing**
- Assume that an emergency will happen.
- Assume that the emergency will be as bad as it can get.
- Develop an emergency communication plan in advance – this will dramatically increase your ability to respond to the unexpected.
- Develop messages and background materials in advance.
- Form strong links with partners, stakeholders and the media well ahead of time – investing in their cooperation will prove invaluable.

# STEP 5: Identify media outlets and media activities

> **BOX 5.2: ACTIVITY GUIDELINES FOR THE FIRST 24–72 HOURS AFTER NOTIFICATION AND VERIFICATION OF A PUBLIC HEALTH EMERGENCY**
>
> **General**
> - ensure the leadership of the organization is aware of the emergency;
> - activate the media communication plan and team;
> - use the communication plan's notification list to ensure the organization's chain of command is aware that the plan has been activated;
> - provide the leadership with an assessment of the emergency from a media perspective; and
> - inform the leadership of the specific steps being taken to proactively and reactively interact with the media.
>
> **Coordination**
> - contact local, provincial, regional, national and international partners using predetermined contact lists;
> - add names and organizations to the contact list as appropriate, based on the event;
> - seek to arrange face-to-face meetings with partners;
> - if a crime may have been committed, contact law-enforcement partners;
> - activate the lead media spokespersons as designated in the media communication plan;
> - call in extra media communication staff in line with the media communication plan;
> - establish roles and responsibilities; and
> - contact public information officers from all responding organizations.
>
> **Media**
> - provide a statement that shows that the organization is aware of the emergency and that details the steps being taken;
> - give directions to the media on how to obtain updates; and
> - start monitoring the media (including the internet) for misinformation and rumours that may need to be corrected.
>
> **Public**
> - activate the public information response system (for example, telephone hotlines) if you anticipate that the public will be seeking information directly from the organization;
> - acknowledge uncertainty;
> - ensure all public statements contain appropriate levels of empathy, caring, concern and compassion, especially regarding losses;
> - provide only facts that have been verified and cleared;
> - refer the public to other information sites, as appropriate;
> - remind the public that the organization has a process in place to respond to the emergency; and
> - start monitoring requests for information to identify trends (**FIGURE EIGHT**).
>
> **Partners and stakeholders**
> - send draft media statements to partners for coordination and, if needed, approval;
> - use pre-arranged notification systems to alert partners;
> - engage the leadership to make important phone calls to partners and leaders of key stakeholder organizations;
> - use the internal organizational communication system to notify employees of the emergency;
> - ask employees for their support;
> - assign tasks to team members, and set hours of operation accordingly; and
> - establish a location from which you can conduct joint operations – for example, a multi-agency Joint Information Centre (JIC).
>
> *These guidelines should be adapted to meet local needs*

## FIGURE EIGHT: WORKSHEET FOR TRACKING ENQUIRIES WITHIN THE FIRST 24–72 HOURS OF AN EMERGENCY

Time of enquiry: _____

Nature of enquiry: _____

Specific information requested:

a. Topic 1: _____
b. Topic 2: _____
c. Topic 3: _____
d. Topic 4: _____

Type of enquiry:

a. For information (if so, what): _____
b. For recommendation (if so, what): _____
c. For action (if so, what): _____
d. Other: _____

Feedback to leadership:

a. Complaint: _____
b. Rumour: _____
c. Misinformation: _____
d. Other: _____

Outcome of call:

a. Able to respond to person: _____
b. Not able to respond to person: _____
c. Referred person to: _____
d. Other: _____

Further action needed:

a. None: _____
b. Provide further information: _____
c. Return call: _____

Urgency level (Check one):

_____ Critical (respond immediately)

_____ Urgent (respond within 24 hours or less)

_____ Routine

Enquiry taken by: _____

Date: _____

This form should be adapted to meet local needs

# STEP 6
## Deliver messages

**6.1:** *Deliver* clear and timely messages
**6.2:** *Deliver* messages to maintain visibility
**6.3:** *Deliver* targeted messages

# STEP 6
## Deliver messages

**6.1:** *Deliver* clear and timely messages
**6.2:** *Deliver* messages to maintain visibility
**6.3:** *Deliver* targeted messages

# 6.1: DELIVER CLEAR AND TIMELY MESSAGES

At the start of an emergency it is important to be able to quickly turn to the prepared media communication plan and to rely the approach it sets out. A sound communication plan helps an organization to proceed confidently and to quickly establish its leadership and trust credentials. In terms of message delivery, it is very important to be:

- first;
- accurate;
- honest;
- accessible;
- credible;
- willing and able to correct misinformation and quell rumours;
- consistent;
- appropriate;
- regular; and
- relevant.

Getting the overarching message across to the intended audience is the ultimate aim of message-delivery activities. During media exchanges it is crucially important to focus on a few key messages that are timely, accurate, clear, concise, credible and memorable. One technique for ensuring this is to use "bridging statements" that link one message to another (**BOX 6.1**). Such bridging is a powerful means of gaining back control during interactions with reporters. If done well, bridging significantly increases the probability that the key messages will appear in the final story. By using bridging techniques, a spokesperson can focus the interview on what is most important, relevant and critical. It also gives the spokesperson a strong sense of control and ownership.

## I. Questions for assessing delivery performance

### 1. Understandability, clarity and brevity

- Did you deliver information in a clear manner?
- Was the language you used appropriate for your target audience?
- Did you tell your audience what you wanted them to know, tell them more and tell them again?
- Were your sentences short?
- Did you avoid the use of undefined jargon, acronyms and technical language that would not be understood by your target audience?
- Did you focus on only 3 messages or pieces of information at a time?
- Did you state your message as a media sound bite (3 messages in less than 27 words and less than 9 seconds)?
- Did you provide supporting facts for your key messages?
- Did you bridge to your key messages using bridging statements?
- Did you support your message with anecdotes and human-interest stories?
- Did you use examples to illustrate and clarify what you are saying?

## 2. IDK ("I don't know")

- When confronted with a question which you could not (or would not) answer, did you say, "I wish I could answer that, however…" or "I don't know" or "I can't answer that"?
- Did you provide a valid reason for not answering the question?
- Did you provide follow-up actions or access to other sources of information?
- Did you give a deadline for follow-up actions?
- Did you bridge to information you could talk about factually?
- Did you repeat the question?

## 3. Interrogation (for example, when asked the same question several times)

- Did you repeat your first answer and indicate that you were repeating it?
- On the second repetition, did you indicate that you had already answered the question and would like to move on to another topic, or were willing to go into more detail?
- On the third repetition, did you indicate that you had answered the question and, if there were no additional questions, did you bridge to another topic or end the interaction?

## 4. First and last

- For any list, did you provide the most important items first and last?

## 5. Trust and CCO (compassion; conviction; optimism)

- When responding to a question or comment about loss of any kind (including death or injury) did you first express compassion, empathy, caring or listening?
- Did you display verbal and non-verbal listening skills?
- Did you avoid criticizing anyone who would have higher credibility than you with your target audience?
- Did you act in partnership with credible third parties?
- Did you identify in your answers support or endorsement from credible third parties or other information sources (for example, scientific journals)?

## 6. Negatives – 1N=3P (one negative equals three positives)

- Did you avoid repeating a negative or false allegation?
- In response to false negatives, criticisms or allegations, did you provide at least three opposing positive, solution-oriented or constructive statements?

## 7. Absolutes

- Did you avoid providing unqualified or unnecessary absolutes (such as the words always, no, not, never, nothing and none)?
- Did you avoid providing over-reassurance that went beyond the facts?
- Did you provide information that gives people a sense of control (for example, by giving people something to do)?

## 8. Non-verbal communication

- Did your non-verbal communication contribute to your message (eyes, hands, dress, posture and room arrangement)?
- Did you avoid fidgeting, engaging in repetitive motions or otherwise displaying distracting body language?

## 9. Visuals

- Did you support and reinforce your message with visual aids such as graphics, charts, maps, timelines, diagrams, photographs, props, flowcharts, checklists, animation or video clips?

## 10. Key messages

- Did you have an overarching (core/key) message set (3 messages totalling 27 words or fewer)?
- Did you repeat and bridge to your key messages at opportune times?
- Did you provide guidance on where to obtain additional information that expands on your key messages?

## 11. Media

- Did you ask about, discuss and agree upon the subject of the interview in advance?
- Did you ask about the questions that might be asked?
- Did you negotiate the length and duration of the interview?
- Did you negotiate the timing of the interview?
- Did you negotiate other aspects of the interview before beginning (such as logistics, including who would do the interview)?
- Did you avoid speaking off-the-record or outside your prepared remarks?
- Did you maintain your composure?
- Did you avoid saying "no comment" or the equivalent to a question?
- Did you acknowledge uncertainty?
- Did you avoid going beyond the bounds of your responsibilities (for example, by speaking for others)?
- Did you avoid using costs as an excuse for not taking an action?
- Did you act at all times as if you were on-camera and on-the-record?
- Did you refrain from using inappropriate humour?

## 12. Pitfalls and opportunities

- Did you use numbers, statistics and data effectively?
- Did you allow yourself to be intimidated by a reporter who used silence as a means to get you to go beyond your message points?
- Did you avoid guessing about facts of which you were unsure?

### BOX 6.1: THE 33 MOST FREQUENTLY USED BRIDGING STATEMENTS

1. And what's most important to know is…
2. However, what is more important to look at is…
3. However, the real issue here is…
4. And what this all means is…
5. And what's most important to remember is…
6. With this in mind, if we look at the bigger picture…
7. With this in mind, if we take a look back…
8. If we take a broader perspective…
9. If we look at the big picture…
10. Let me put all this in perspective by saying…
11. What all this information tells me is…
12. Before we continue, let me take a step back and repeat that…
13. Before we continue, let me emphasize that…
14. This is an important point because…
15. What this all boils down to is…
16. The heart of the matter is…
17. What matters most in this situation is…
18. And as I said before…
19. And if we take a closer look, we would see…
20. Let me just add to this that…
21. I think it would be more correct to say…
22. Let me point out again that…
23. Let me emphasize again…
24. In this context, it is essential that I note…
25. Another thing to remember is…
26. Before we leave the subject, let me add that…
27. And that reminds me…
28. And the one thing that is important to remember is…
29. What I've said comes down to this…
30. Here's the real issue…
31. While… is important, it is also important to remember…
32. It's true that… but it is also true that…
33. What is key here is…

# 6.2: DELIVER MESSAGES TO MAINTAIN VISIBILITY

Time is precious during an emergency, and delays in acquiring and distributing sound information can be very difficult to overcome. As a result, other (possibly less trustworthy) sources may move to fill the information voids. Do not wait – it is better to come out early and say that information is preliminary and that updates will be forthcoming. The key activity points at this time include:

- brief the media promptly following an incident;
- fill information voids;
- state, if appropriate, that the information is preliminary;
- acknowledge uncertainty;
- state that the media will be updated promptly as additional information becomes available;
- state what is factual, what is known and what is not known;
- avoid speculation;
- hold regular briefings;
- correct misconceptions or misinformation already in the public domain;
- state when you expect new information to become available;
- if the situation warrants it, provide hotlines and telephone information services for the media, the public and special groups (for example, nurses, doctors and other health professionals) – make sure there are enough people to answer the telephone calls;
- provide a media communication centre staffed 24 hours per day; and
- plan how often you will provide information updates, who will do it and how.

## I. Informational events to promote visibility

Typical informational events to promote visibility include:

### 1. News conferences

News conferences are held to provide journalists with information on an issue. A news conference is also a good way to provide journalists with an update of key developments and with information on an organization's plans, work and policies. News conferences are the most common media event during an emergency. As with all media events, it is best to plan them in advance, even if they are only minutes or hours away. A news conference is typically held to announce a major event, decision or news item (such as the release of a report, a new policy, a policy change or the announcement of an actual emergency). They can also be used to draw attention to a particular public health issue.

### 2. Town meetings

Town meetings are held during and after an emergency, and are often very difficult to do well. The standard format for many town meetings is to have officials and experts sit in the front of the room (often behind a long table) facing the audience (for example, members of the affected community or the families of victims). Town meetings must be carefully planned as they can potentially become uncontrollable and sometimes riotous. The media frequently focus on negative or emotion-laden comments made at town meetings.

## 3. Informational meetings

Informational meetings include open houses, information exchanges and expert availability sessions, and are less of a media event and more of an opportunity to provide information face-to-face with key stakeholders. They can be a good opportunity to exchange information. However, because of logistical problems, they are seldom used in the acute phase of an emergency.

## 4. Media availability sessions

Media availability sessions are typically used to bring spokespersons from partner organizations together in person or on the telephone for questioning by the media. Media availability sessions ensure that partners hear each other's responses to questions from the media. They reduce the chances that one partner will be played off against the other.

# II. News conferences

Of the informational events described above, news conferences are often the most important events during an emergency. News conferences can be major undertakings and often require much work and preparation to be successful. You should consider dividing the work among staff members to make planning easier.

## 1. Location of a news conference

- find a well-known location convenient for journalists – if you don't have an appropriate site in your office building, popular sites for media events include hotels, local press clubs and public buildings in a centralized location;
- make sure the room is not too large otherwise there may be a lot of empty seats, giving the impression that few journalists attended;
- make sure however that there is sufficient room and places for all the speakers to stand or sit (for example, a long table or sufficient space behind the podium for the speakers to stand);
- ensure that there is adequate open space for television cameras, lights and microphones;
- provide technical support and seating convenient for different media (such as forward seating for radio);
- if resources allow, provide access to the internet (for example through wireless connections or dedicated computers); and
- ensure there are an adequate number of electrical outlets.

## 2. Timing of a news conference

- remember that journalists have busy schedules;
- because of deadlines, often the best time to hold a media event is around 10:00–11:00 hrs on a weekday morning or 15:00–16:00 hrs on a weekday afternoon – although this may vary by country or locality;
- plan around competing events and other activities that may prevent journalists from attending the event;
- in fast-breaking emergencies, consider holding at least two news conferences per day (thereby allowing the spokesperson to gather more information, to come back the same day to give more in-depth information, and to say: "I don't know the answer to that now but I will try to have more information for you later today);
- accommodate local and national media deadlines; and
- never delay the release of critical information.

## 3. Contacting the media about a news conference
- send a media advisory in advance by post if time allows – otherwise email or fax the advisory;
- include in the advisory:
  - the location
  - the start and finish times
  - the date
  - a brief description of what will be covered
  - names and titles of speakers;
- bear in mind that newsrooms are often swamped with releases, faxes and invitations to events; and
- be considerate of the reporter's time when scheduling media events when no new information is to be reported.

## 4. Materials for a news conference
- put together a media kit, media packet or other information materials to give to journalists attending the event;
- consider handing out a page at the outset of the session with the names, titles and responsibilities of the presenters;
- make sure you have plenty of copies of media packets or information materials in case more people attend than expected;
- provide resources for out-of-town media, such as maps of the area showing hotels and restaurants; and
- have a sign-in sheet for journalists attending, and use this sheet to update your media contact list.

> **INFORMATION POINT: Contents of a media kit or packet**
> - news releases;
> - fact sheets;
> - biographies of speakers, subject-matter experts and others as appropriate;
> - contact numbers;
> - copies of any reports or documents that would be useful to reporters covering the event;
> - visual material (such as maps, charts, timelines, diagrams, drawings and photographs); and
> - other materials as appropriate.

## 5. Preparations for a news conference
- set up the room for the number of people you invited;
- set up a podium, if appropriate;
- don't be disappointed if fewer people show up than expected – attendance is hard to predict;
- have staff available to assist journalists before, during and after the event;
- have someone help with the handing out of media kits or packets, managing the sign-in sheet, directing journalists to telephones and handling any last-minute details;
- select a moderator for the event who will set the ground rules, such as:
  - all reporters asking a question must first be recognized by the moderator
  - each reporter recognized by the moderator will be allowed to ask one question and one follow-up question
  - all questions should be directed to the moderator who in turn will direct the question to the appropriate speaker
  - reporters should indicate which speaker they would like to answer the question;

STEP 6: Deliver messages

- determine beforehand who will make the opening remarks and introduce each speaker;
- set ground rules for camera placement and movement during the event;
- supply the necessary lighting and audio (microphone) hook-ups for electronic media;
- develop anticipated questions and answers for speakers; and
- rehearse the speakers if possible, asking them basic and difficult questions.

> **INFORMATION POINT: Holding a news conference**
>
> - Make your formal opening statement brief – around 5 minutes and definitely less than 10 minutes.
> - Make sure you mention all pertinent information (for example, who, what, where, when, why and how) in your opening statement.
> - Allow time for questions (typically at least 10–15 minutes).
> - As a general rule, limit the number of speakers to no more than three.
> - If additional people are available to answer questions, have them sit in the front row or off to the side.
> - As a general rule, limit each speaker to no more than 5 minutes.
> - Start on time – journalists work to deadlines and need time to complete their story in time.
> - Remember that a news conference is held primarily to allow the media to ask questions, not attend a lecture.

## 6. Follow-up to a news conference

- thank reporters for attending;
- allow time at the conclusion of the event to arrange photographs;
- tell reporters how unanswered questions raised in the news conference will be handled and provide call-in number or web-site information;
- tell reporters when the next news conference will be held, if one is scheduled;
- offer to fax or email materials to those journalists who were unable to attend;
- make sure your staff knows where to direct telephone calls from journalists calling after the event;
- monitor media coverage;
- recognize that reporters and editors often pay attention to letters (both positive and negative) about news stories and may integrate the comments into future stories; and
- correct any significant errors in reporting in accordance with the process outlined in **BOX 6.2**.

> **BOX 6.2: CORRECTING ERRORS IN MEDIA REPORTING**
>
> **If there is an error in the story:**
>
> - Remain calm and composed when speaking to reporters or editors about errors and mistakes.
> - Contact the reporter directly and point out errors only if the errors are significant.
> - Do not complain about trivial mistakes or omissions.
> - Ask the reporter to amend the office file copy of the story.
> - Consider asking the reporter to make an appropriate change in their next story – note however that this can be controversial and lead to a difficult relationship with the journalist.
> - Avoid embarrassing the reporter by naming them during a news or press conference or briefing.
> - Avoid if possible going to the reporter's editor or producer – this should only be done if there is a major mistake, and if the reporter will not acknowledge the mistake and make the requested correction. By going over the reporter's head, you may ruin any working relationship you have developed.
> - If the error occurs in the stories of several different reporters, or if the story is picked up by a wire service, and if the error is deemed major, then correct the error during the next news release, media briefing or news conference without naming the individuals responsible for the error.
> - Recognize the difference between errors and differences in points of view – differences in points of view will generally not be corrected.

# 6.3: DELIVER TARGETED MESSAGES

## I. Strategies for delivering targeted messages

Cooperation from the media is often needed to deliver targeted public health messages during an emergency. Journalists, however, may have different interests and may not assign the same priority as public health officials to such messages. As a result, public health officials must engage in special efforts to make their messages more interesting, relevant and attractive both to the media and to the target audience (**BOX 6.3**).

---

**BOX 6.3: STRATEGIES FOR DELIVERING TARGETED MESSAGES**

**To communicate voluntariness – deliver messages that:**
- make the risk more voluntary;
- encourage public dialogue by using two-way communication channels;
- ask permission; and
- ask for informed consent.

**To communicate controllability – deliver messages that:**
- identify things for people to do (for example, precautions, preventive actions and treatments);
- indicate your willingness to cooperate and share authority and responsibility with others;
- give important roles and responsibilities to others;
- tell people how to recognize problems or symptoms; and
- tell people how and where to get further information.

**To communicate familiarity – deliver messages that:**
- use analogies to make the unfamiliar familiar;
- have a strong visual content; and
- describe means for exploring issues in greater depth.

**To communicate fairness – deliver messages that:**
- acknowledge possible inequities;
- address inequities; and
- discuss options and trade-offs.

**To communicate trust – deliver messages that:**
- cite credible third parties;
- cite credible sources for further information;
- acknowledge that there are other points of view;
- indicate a willingness to be held accountable;
- describe achievements;
- indicate conformance with the highest professional, scientific and ethical standards;
- cite scientific research – be prepared to point to specific published studies;
- describe the review, approval and advisory processes;
- identify the partners working with you; and
- indicate your willingness to share the risk ("do unto others only that which you would be willing to do unto yourself or your loved ones").

## II. Strategies for enhancing delivery

One of the first steps in delivering targeted and effective messages is to find out what the reporter needs and wants. One way of achieving this is to ask the reporter a series of questions – both topic-related (**BOX 6.4**) and procedural (**BOX 6.5**) – before the interview. The most important of these will be:

### 1. What is the subject or topic of the interview?

It is your right to ask this question and to receive a reasonable response. The answer to this question will be crucial in:

- establishing what the reporter wants;
- deciding if you are the right person to be interviewed;
- establishing a verbal contract with the reporter regarding the boundaries of the interview that can be called upon if needed during or after the interview; and
- deciding what your key messages will be.

> **BOX 6.4: EXAMPLES OF TOPIC-RELATED QUESTIONS TO ASK A REPORTER BEFORE A MEDIA INTERVIEW**
>
> Answers to the following topic-related questions can provide valuable information. However, time is seldom available, especially during an emergency, to ask them all. In addition, reporters may find some questions – particularly those marked below with an * – offensive, insulting or inappropriate for a news source to ask. The following list should be reviewed and judgement exercised in selecting 3–4 questions appropriate to the situation, available time and specific reporter.
>
> - What is the subject or topic of the interview?
> - What is the focus of the interview?
> - What specific subjects does the reporter expect to cover in the interview?
> - What is the most important thing that the reporter would like to know? Would the reporter like to receive background material related to the topic before conducting the interview?
> - Would the reporter like suggestions about who else to interview?
> - If you are not the right person for the interview, would the reporter like suggestions about who would be better?
> - What types of questions will be asked?*
> - What specific questions will be asked?*
> - Has the reporter done any background research related to the topic of the interview?*
> - If so, what was found and where?*
> - Who else has the reporter interviewed?*
> - What did they say?*
> - Who else does the reporter expect to interview for the story?*
> - How will the reporter use the interview material?*
> - How will the interview material fit into the story?*

### 2. Timing of an interview

Timing is crucial during an emergency. Time pressures and anxiety levels will be extremely high. Late messages are often ineffective and so delaying can mean losing the initiative. Within the limits of privacy, security and other laws, regulations or policies, it is therefore extremely important to provide journalists with all the available verified and cleared information quickly and on time.

> **BOX 6.5: EXAMPLES OF PROCEDURAL QUESTIONS TO ASK A REPORTER BEFORE A MEDIA INTERVIEW**
>
> Answers to procedural questions can provide valuable information. However, as with topic-related questions, time is seldom available (especially during an emergency) to ask them all. In addition, reporters may find some of the following questions – particularly those marked below with as asterisk (*) – offensive, insulting or inappropriate for a news source to ask. The following list should be reviewed and judgement exercised in selecting 3–4 questions appropriate to the situation, available time and the specific reporter.
>
> **Background questions**
> - Who will be conducting the interview?
> - What is the reporter's name, media affiliation, telephone number, cell/mobile phone number, fax number and email address?
> - Is the reporter a staff member (full-time or part-time) or a freelancer?
> - Does the reporter specialize in any particular area?
> - What type of publication or programme is it?
> - When will the story be published or broadcast?
> - Who generally reads, sees or hears the publication or programme?
> - What stories have previously been covered by the reporter?*
> - How long has the reporter been a journalist?*
> - Will the reporter have any say in writing the headline or the lead for the story?*
>
> **Logistical questions**
> - What is the reporter's deadline for the story?
> - Is the reporter's deadline flexible?
> - Will it be possible for the interviewee to get back to the reporter to do the interview later?
> - If so, when?
> - Where will the interview take place?
> - How long will the interview take?
> - What is the format for the interview – for example, live, tape, sit-down, stand-up or panel?
> - Can the interviewee use notes?
> - Who else will be present at the interview?
> - Will there be other reporters or guests?
> - Will the interview be audio recorded or videotaped by the reporter?
> - Where will the story appear (for example, will it be the lead story)?*
> - Is the story likely to appear elsewhere?*
> - If so, where?*
> - How long will the story be?*
> - How many seconds/words will be taken from the interview for the story?*
> - Does the reporter call back to verify the accuracy of specific quotes attributed directly to the person being interviewed?*
> - Will the person being interviewed be allowed to have an input regarding interview setting, such as seating arrangements?*
> - If the interview will be audio recorded or videotaped by the reporter, can a copy be made available for archiving?*
> - Will it be acceptable if the interviewee records the interview?*

## 3. After the interview

Even after the interview is over, several useful things can still be done:

- **Conclusion** – when asked at the end of the interview if you would like to add anything more, repeat your primary key messages.
- **Follow-up** – indicate your willingness to be available if additional questions arise related to technical issues or the story.
- **Recording and archiving** – you can request a taped copy or written transcript of the programme or publication for your files. If you provide a videocassette or audiocassette prior to the programme, they may make a tape for you. When time permits, review the tape with a media specialist to identify ways of improving future performance. If the situation warrants, send a thank you note.

# STEP 7
## Evaluate messages and performance

**7.1:** *Evaluate* message delivery and media coverage

**7.2:** *Evaluate* and improve performance based on feedback

**7.3:** *Evaluate* public responses to messages

# STEP 7
## Evaluate messages and performance

**7.1:** *Evaluate* message delivery and media coverage

**7.2:** *Evaluate* and improve performance based on feedback

**7.3:** *Evaluate* public responses to messages

# 7.1: EVALUATE MESSAGE DELIVERY AND MEDIA COVERAGE

## I. Evaluating message delivery

**BOXES 7.1–7.3** present a list of measures that can be used to evaluate the likely success or otherwise of message delivery in terms of:

- the openness and transparency of communications;
- the use of listening techniques; and
- message clarity.

### BOX 7.1: EVALUATING OPENNESS AND TRANSPARENCY OF COMMUNICATIONS

- Were you candid and open with reporters?
- Were you the first to reveal bad news?
- If the answer to a question was unknown or uncertain, did you express willingness to get back to the reporter with a response within an agreed upon deadline (assuming the story was not reported in real time)?
- If you were in doubt, did you lean towards sharing more information not less?
- Were you especially careful when asked to speculate or answer "what if" questions, especially about worst-case scenarios?

**Did you:**

- disclose risk information as soon as possible (emphasizing appropriate reservations about reliability)?
- fill information vacuums?
- minimize or exaggerate the level of risk? Over reassure?
- make corrections quickly if errors were made?
- discuss data and information uncertainties, strengths and weaknesses – including those identified by other credible sources?
- identify worst-case estimates as such, and cite ranges of risk estimates when appropriate?
- tell the truth?

## BOX 7.2: EVALUATING LISTENING

Did you:

- target the right audience?
- miss listening to anybody important (stakeholders or partners)?
- avoid making assumptions about what viewers, listeners and readers knew, thought or wanted done about the risks or the situation?
- identify with the target audience and try empathetically to put yourself in their place?
- acknowledge the validity of people's emotions and fears?
- respond (in words, gestures and actions) to emotions that people expressed, such as anxiety, fear, anger, outrage and helplessness?
- express genuine empathy when responding to questions about loss?
- acknowledge, and say, that any illness, injury or death is a tragedy?
- use media outlets that encourage listening, feedback, participation and dialogue?
- avoid distant, abstract and unfeeling language about harm, deaths, injuries and illnesses?
- recognize that competing agendas, symbolic meanings, and broader social, cultural, economic or political considerations often complicate the task of effective media communication?
- display sensitivity to local norms, such as in speech and dress?
- review available data and information on what people were thinking before media interviews?
  Examples include data and information drawn from interviews, facilitated discussion groups, public meetings, public hearings, information exchanges, availability sessions, advisory groups, logs from hotlines or toll-free numbers, and surveys.

## BOX 7.3: EVALUATING CLARITY

Did you:

- speak at the appropriate level of comprehension for your target audience?
- keep your sentences short and focused?
- use clear, non-technical language?
- use graphics and visual aids to clarify messages?
- respect the unique media communication needs of special and diverse audiences?
- translate and test messages to meet the cultural and language needs of special populations?
- consider how best to express messages intended to have global reach?
- personalize risk data?
- use examples and anecdotes that made data come alive?
- acknowledge and respond to the distinctions that the public views as important in evaluating risks?
- use risk comparisons to help put risks in perspective, and avoid comparisons that ignored the distinctions people consider important?
- identify specific actions that people can take to protect themselves and to maintain control of the situation at hand?
- strive for brevity?
- offer to provide needed additional information within the reporter's deadline?
- provide the reporter with information about actions that were under way or that could be taken?
- promise only that which could be delivered and then follow through?

## II. Evaluating media coverage

**BOX 7.4** presents measures to evaluate the success or otherwise of activities aimed at achieving newspaper, radio, television and internet coverage during an emergency. These measures could also be applied to smaller scale approaches such as traditional and folk media. Most of the measures are *process* evaluation measures, not outcome evaluation measures (**BOX 7.5**). They provide information only on the media coverage achieved not on the impact made on the target audience.

## BOX 7.4: EVALUATION OF MEDIA COVERAGE

### Newspapers
- How many newspapers published or carried your information?
- How many published or carried the information of other organizations? Did the information reinforce your message or was it competitive?
- How prominent were the articles – front page; above the "fold"?
- Did the articles convey your messages without distortion?

### Radio
- How many radio spots, news items or mentions resulted from your message?
- What were the audience ratings data?
- How many radio spots, news items or mentions resulted from the messages of other organizations? Did the information reinforce your messages or was it competitive?
- Were the radio spots transmitted at peak listening times?
- Were your remarks edited appropriately?
- Were you successful in getting across your key messages and "sound bites"?
- Were other organizations successful in getting across their key messages and "sound bites"?

### Television
- How many television spots, news items or mentions resulted from your messages?
- What were the audience ratings data?
- How many television spots, news items or mentions resulted from the messages of other organizations?
- Were the television spots transmitted at peak listening time?
- Were you edited appropriately?
- Were you successful in getting across your key messages and "sound bites"?
- Were other organizations successful in getting across their key messages and "sound bites"? Did the information reinforce your message or was it competitive?

### Internet
- How many visits ("hits") did your organizational web site receive?
- Were your messages quoted or mentioned on the web sites of other organizations?
- Were the messages of individuals or organizations with an opposing viewpoint quoted or mentioned on the web sites of other organizations?
- Were you quoted or edited accurately and appropriately?
- Were you successful in getting across your key messages and "sound bites"?
- How many "counter sites" offered other or opposing viewpoints?
- Were other organizations successful in getting across their key messages and "sound bites"? Did the information reinforce your message or was it competitive?

## BOX 7.5: TYPES OF EVALUATION

There are two basic types of evaluation:

### 1. Process evaluation

Process evaluation tracks progress and is typically used to:
- track how well media communication activities are working; and
- assess administrative and organizational aspects of media communication activities.

For example, if the communication plan includes a toll-free number, a mechanism can be established (such as a simple response form) to record the questions that are asked and the answers that are given. Reviews of these responses will reveal whether or not:
- correct or adequate information is being given;
- new information is needed to respond adequately; and
- there is any pattern to the questions.

### 2. Outcome evaluation

Outcome evaluation is used to measure programme effectiveness by demonstrating what (if any) objectives were accomplished. Outcome evaluation encompasses and goes beyond process evaluation and provides valuable information on the value of communication activities. This can include assessing whether or not the target audience learned, acted or made changes as a result of communications.

Outcome evaluation typically involves before-and-after comparisons. For example, comparing target audience awareness or attitudes before and after one or more communication activities. Outcome evaluation measures can also be observational or self-reported (for example, interviews with members of the target audience). Despite its value, systematic and comprehensive outcome evaluation is seldom undertaken due to:
- limited funds;
- limited time;
- limited capabilities;
- the need to return to daily duties;
- organizational and bureaucratic constraints; and
- difficulties in designing appropriate measures of success or effectiveness.

## INFORMATION POINT: Examples of process evaluation measures

- time schedules;
- expenditures;
- work performed;
- volume of enquiries from the public (for example, through analysis of telephone hotline call-in logs);
- fact sheets distributed; and
- participation by the target audience in communication activities (for example, the number of journalists who attended a media event).

## INFORMATION POINT: Examples of outcome evaluation measures

**Changes in:**
- knowledge;
- understanding;
- awareness;
- cooperation;
- support for policies or plans;
- attitudes;
- opinions;
- beliefs;
- decisions; and
- trust in health authorities.

## 7.2: EVALUATE AND IMPROVE PERFORMANCE BASED ON FEEDBACK

Performance improvement requires performance evaluation to help identify the gaps and deficiencies to be addressed and corrected. Based on the results of evaluation, changes can be made to ensure the achievement of goals and objectives. Although evaluation is identified in this handbook as the final linear step in media communication, in reality it is an ongoing and nearly continuous process. The true final step in ensuring effective media communication during public health emergencies is to close the seven-step loop by reviewing and then improving all communication plans, strategies and messages based on feedback. Each step in media communication can be subjected to evaluation, and lessons learned for all subsequent activities. **BOXES 7.6–7.10** present a number of key activity areas in which the performance of the communication system can be can be rapidly assessed.

### BOX 7.6: EVALUATING SYSTEM PERFORMANCE – MEDIA COMMUNICATION PLANNING

**Did you:**

- begin the media-planning effort with clear, explicit objectives – such as providing information, establishing trust, encouraging appropriate actions, stimulating emergency responses or involving stakeholders in dialogue, partnerships and joint problem-solving?
- assess media needs and organize ways to meet these needs?
- identify important stakeholders and subgroups within the audience as targets for your media messages?
- identify credible third parties who could support your messages?
- train staff in media-communication skills and in public health?
- recruit lead media spokespersons with effective presentation and personal-interaction skills?
- recognize and reward outstanding media performance?
- anticipate questions and issues that might be raised in an interview?
- set up a system to monitor what appeared on web sites and other online media?
- prepare and pre-test messages before offering them to the media?
- set up a system for practising media interviews?
- determine who would conduct media briefings?
- set up a system to confirm facts?
- establish an organizational protocol for all contacts with the media?
- ensure that all staff were aware of the organizational protocol for all contact with the media?
- establish an efficient clearance and approval procedure for all messages intended for the media?
- ensure that all staff were aware of the formal clearance procedure for all messages intended for the media?
- ensure that all staff were aware of policies regarding media contacts?
- rehearse with your lead media spokesperson prior to media contact?
- determine how you would greet, register and handle reporters who arrived on site?
- develop a triage system for prioritizing and responding to media requests and enquiries?
- develop media contact lists?
- carefully evaluate media-communication efforts and learn from mistakes?
- share with others what you have learned from working with the media in an emergency?

### STEP 7: Evaluate messages and performance

> **BOX 7.7: EVALUATING SYSTEM PERFORMANCE – WORKING WITH THE MEDIA AND MEETING THE MEDIA'S FUNCTIONAL NEEDS**
>
> **Working with the media**
>
> **Did you:**
>
> - keep the media well informed of decisions and actions?
> - avoid being defensive or argumentative in interviews?
> - include in interviews, factors that make a story interesting to the media, including factors that influence public perceptions of risk?
> - strive for "win-win" media outcomes?
>
> **Were you:**
>
> - accessible to reporters?
> - polite and courteous at all times, even if the reporter was not?
>
> **Meeting the functional needs of the media**
>
> **Did you:**
>
> - meet the media's functional needs – for example, by providing information tailored to the needs of each type of media, such as sound bites, background videotape and other visual materials for television?
> - provide information to the media that recognized and met their deadlines?
> - provide the media with timely, accurate, clear and credible press releases, media alerts, press statements, fact sheets and question and answer (Q&A) sheets?
> - anticipate the questions that the media would ask?
> - prepare a limited number of key messages in advance of media interactions?
> - repeat your key messages several times?
> - provide background materials for reporters on complex risk or public-health issues?
> - prepare background video for television use?
> - offer reporters the opportunity to interview spokespersons one-on-one at media availability sessions?
> - keep media interviews short?
> - agree with the reporter in advance about logistics, including the specific topic of the interview?
> - stick to the agreed topic during the interview?
> - bridge to important messages to bring the interview back on track?
> - offer to follow-up on questions that could not be addressed immediately?
> - offer follow-up contact information?
> - avoid saying "no comment"?
> - work to establish relationships with reporters and editors prior to the emergency?
> - meet with reporters who would cover the story before the event occurred?
> - create a log of media calls?
> - focus on what you do know, and tell the reporter what actions you would be willing to take if you did not know the answer to a question?
> - exercise extreme caution in going "off the record" or providing "background" information?

### BOX 7.8: EVALUATING SYSTEM PERFORMANCE – COORDINATION ACTIVITIES

**Did you (to the extent feasible):**

- work with partner organizations in developing consistent messages?
- coordinate communications within and across agencies, especially before media briefings, news conferences and media interviews?
- contact partner organizations to let them know the actions being taken?
- distribute your communication materials to partner organizations?
- offer to conduct special briefings for partner organizations?
- offer other organizations the opportunity to conduct joint briefings for the media?
- devote effort and resources to building bridges, relationships, partnerships and alliances with partner organizations before an emergency occurred?
- consult with partner organizations to determine who should take the lead in responding to media enquiries in various scenarios or on various topics concerning the emergency?
- document all agreements with partner organizations?
- maintain credibility by not criticizing individuals or organizations with higher perceived credibility?
- cite credible and authoritative sources that believe what you believe?
- issue media communications together with, or through, other trustworthy sources?

### BOX 7.9: EVALUATING SYSTEM PERFORMANCE – MEDIA AND OUTREACH TASKS

**Media tasks**

**Did you:**

- organize news briefings?
- produce and distribute news releases?
- respond to media requests and enquiries?
- provide support for spokespersons?
- conduct news conferences?

**Outreach tasks**

**Did you:**

- coordinate and maintain contact with governmental, nongovernmental, not-for-profit, and private-sector organizations?
- distribute informational materials contained in the media kit or packet in advance to partner organizations?
- coordinate public-service announcements and public-education campaigns?

## BOX 7.10: EVALUATING SYSTEM PERFORMANCE – HOTLINES AND WEB SITES

**Hotlines**

**Did you:**

- brief hotline operators on how to respond to calls from the public?
- provide hotline operations with a list of frequently asked questions (FAQs)?
- provide hotline operators with scripts for responding to frequently asked questions?
- provide guidance to hotline operators on how to use scripts when responding to calls?
- report back on results from hotline calls to others members of the communication team?
- update the communication team on callers' questions for which you did not have answers?

**Web sites**

**Did you:**

- develop content to put on the organization web site in the event of an emergency?
- put information on the web site in a timely manner?
- include content consistent with how web sites are used?
- make sure everything put on the web site had gone through the approval and clearance process?
- create links to other web sites that also had information on the emergency?
- update your web site as information changed?
- provide information to partner organizations for their web sites?

# 7.3: EVALUATE PUBLIC RESPONSES TO MESSAGES

Evaluating public responses to messages requires information from the following categories:

## I. Outreach – how many people were actually reached?

- numbers of communication materials distributed;
- numbers of speeches, presentations, briefings or press conferences conducted;
- size of audiences reached, including numbers of readers, listeners and viewers;
- number of other organizations and persons contacted; and
- number of media outlets covering the story.

## II. Evaluating response – did audiences respond?

- number of enquiries, names or affiliations of those who made enquires, and what they asked;
- drop-off or increase in calls following the start of the information campaign; and
- number of partner organizations, names of partner organizations, and whether or not they cooperated and collaborated.

## III. Evaluating impact – were there changes?

The most important thing to evaluate is the impact of the message on the target audience (**BOX 7.11**). For example, did they hear, understand and act upon what was communicated to them? The overall intention is to gain information so that improvements can be made. Information is gathered and analysed to:

- improve current and future communication efforts;
- verify that change has occurred; and
- identify messages, activities or programmes that are working or not working.

### BOX 7.11: EVALUATING OUTCOME MEASURES

**Were there any before-and-after changes in the following?**

- knowledge;
- attitudes;
- beliefs;
- intentions;
- behaviour; and
- actions.

# ANNEXES

**ANNEX 1.** REFLECTING CULTURAL DIVERSITY IN COMMUNICATION ACTIVITIES AND MATERIALS

**ANNEX 2.** WHO OUTBREAK COMMUNICATION GUIDELINES

**ANNEX 3.** PRINCIPLES AND TECHNIQUES OF EFFECTIVE MEDIA COMMUNICATION

**ANNEX 4.** SAMPLE MEDIA COMMUNICATION PLAN CONTENTS

**ANNEX 5.** SAMPLE LETTER OF ENDORSEMENT BY THE AGENCY DIRECTOR OF THE MEDIA COMMUNICATION PLAN

**ANNEX 6.** QUESTIONS FREQUENTLY ASKED BY JOURNALISTS AND THE PUBLIC DURING DISEASE OUTBREAKS

**ANNEX 7.** EFFECTIVELY COMMUNICATING RISK NUMBERS

**ANNEX 8.** FACTORS IN RISK PERCEPTION

**ANNEX 9.** HOW PEOPLE FORM RISK PERCEPTIONS AND MAKE RISK JUDGEMENTS

**ANNEX 10.** HOW PEOPLE PROCESS RISK INFORMATION IN HIGH-STRESS SITUATIONS

**ANNEX 11.** HOW PEOPLE FORM PERCEPTIONS OF TRUST

# ANNEXES

**ANNEX 1.** REFLECTING CULTURAL DIVERSITY IN COMMUNICATION ACTIVITIES AND MATERIALS

**ANNEX 2.** WHO OUTBREAK COMMUNICATION GUIDELINES

**ANNEX 3.** PRINCIPLES AND TECHNIQUES OF EFFECTIVE MEDIA COMMUNICATION

**ANNEX 4.** SAMPLE MEDIA COMMUNICATION PLAN CONTENTS

**ANNEX 5.** SAMPLE LETTER OF ENDORSEMENT BY THE AGENCY DIRECTOR OF THE MEDIA COMMUNICATION PLAN

**ANNEX 6.** QUESTIONS FREQUENTLY ASKED BY JOURNALISTS AND THE PUBLIC DURING DISEASE OUTBREAKS

**ANNEX 7.** EFFECTIVELY COMMUNICATING RISK NUMBERS

**ANNEX 8.** FACTORS IN RISK PERCEPTION

**ANNEX 9.** HOW PEOPLE FORM RISK PERCEPTIONS AND MAKE RISK JUDGEMENTS

**ANNEX 10.** HOW PEOPLE PROCESS RISK INFORMATION IN HIGH-STRESS SITUATIONS

**ANNEX 11.** HOW PEOPLE FORM PERCEPTIONS OF TRUST

# ANNEX 1. REFLECTING CULTURAL DIVERSITY IN COMMUNICATION ACTIVITIES AND MATERIALS

The WHO Outbreak Communication Guidelines (**ANNEX 2**) were developed to address the common features of communication across many cultures. The guiding principle of effective communication in a global context is that all communication activities and materials (including those prepared for the media) should reflect the diverse nature of societies in a fair, representative and inclusive manner.

## I. Reflecting cultural diversity

### 1. Patterns of cultural difference

To be effective, media communication must be sensitive to cultural differences between and within the various regions and nations of the world. Culture is grounded in a group's shared experience and identity, and in its relationships; both human-to-human and human to animals, objects, gods and the cosmos. Definitions of culture typically include elements such as:

- meanings, interpretations;
- perceptions;
- behaviours;
- language;
- ways of expressing emotions and facts;
- identity;
- assumptions;
- rules, structures and theories for organizing experience;
- ways of interacting;
- beliefs, attitudes;
- thoughts;
- sense of self; and
- religion.

Several of the most important patterns of cultural difference affecting media communications before, during, and after a public health emergency are described below. These differences are a potential source of cross-cultural communication difficulties and must be addressed (**BOX A**).

### 2. Different communication styles

The way people communicate varies widely between and within cultures. One aspect of communication style is language usage. Across cultures, words and phrases are frequently used in different ways. For example, even in countries that share the same language, the meaning of the simple word "yes" varies greatly from: "definitely, I understand what you said" to "maybe" or "I'll consider it", along with many shades in between. Another major aspect of communication style is the degree of importance given to non-verbal communications. Non-verbal communication includes facial expressions and body gestures; it also involves seating arrangements, personal distance, and sense of time. In addition, different norms exist regarding the appropriate degree of assertiveness in communicating information. For instance, some cultures consider raised voices to be threatening or a sign of anger, whereas other cultures consider an increase in volume as a sign of excitement and commitment.

## 3. Different attitudes towards conflict

Some cultures view conflict as a positive aspect of communication, while others view it as something to be avoided. In many cultures, open conflict and disagreements are viewed as embarrassing or demeaning – differences are worked out quietly behind the scenes.

## 4. Different decision-making styles

The roles individuals play in decision-making vary widely from culture to culture:

- In some cultures decisions are frequently delegated – i.e. an official assigns responsibility for a particular matter to a subordinate. In other cultures there is a strong value placed on according decision-making responsibilities to the individual.
- Although individual recognition and initiative are encouraged in some cultures, in others the collective good is emphasized, and individuals are encouraged to sacrifice individual recognition.
- Majority rule is a common approach in many cultures but in other cultures consensus is the preferred mode, or decision-making may be entrusted to an elder or exalted member of the community.

## 5. Different attitudes towards disclosure

In some cultures, it is considered inappropriate to be candid about emotions, about the reasons behind a conflict or a misunderstanding, or about personal information. Questions that may seem natural to one culture may seem intrusive to another.

## 6. Different approaches to knowing

Significant differences occur between cultures in the way people come to "know" things. For example, some cultures consider information acquired through cognitive means (such as counting and measuring) more valid than other, less tangible, ways of knowing (such as intuition).

## 7. Differences in discourse

When communicating with one another, individuals will follow the assumptions and rules governing discourse within their respective cultures. Because significant variations exist in the rules for conversation across different cultures, message design must be sensitive and appropriately tailored. Rules for conversation cover such diverse areas as:

- opening or closing conversations;
- taking turns during conversations;
- interrupting;
- using silence as a communicative device;
- incorporating appropriate topics of conversation or discourse;
- interjecting humour into a conversation;
- using laughter and humour as a communication device;
- using gestures to make or emphasize a point;
- using storytelling and narratives as a communication device;
- speaking for an appropriate amount of time; and
- sequencing of the elements of a speech or conversation.

In some cultures – particularly those with strong oral traditions – people often prefer storytelling and anecdotes as a conversation and communication device. Personal stories and anecdotes are useful tools for bringing information close in time and space to listeners. Stories in this tradition often presume a shared knowledge with the audience, do more showing than telling, imply linkages among a wide range of topics, and contain elements not necessarily presented in temporal sequence.

## 8. Assessing socioeconomic levels

In order to fully inform message design, national, regional, provincial and local socioeconomic levels also need to be taken into account and accurate profiles produced of variables such as:

- income level (for example, mean, median and other characteristics);
- educational level (for example, mean, median and other characteristics); and
- occupation.

Socioeconomic factors affect virtually all communication decisions and choices, including:

- choice of media formats (affected for example by what proportion of the population can read); and
- choice of media technology (affected for example by what proportion of the population own radios, televisions, and land-line and mobile telephones).

> **BOX A: GUIDELINES ON PLANNING AND IMPLEMENTING AN EFFECTIVE AND CULTURALLY SENSITIVE MEDIA PROGRAMME**
>
> Activities and behaviours to be considered when planning and implementing an effective media programme sensitive to the needs of diverse populations include:
> - prepare, produce and disseminate information using diverse forms of media and graphic arts;
> - identify target audiences with special information needs;
> - advocate on behalf of those who will or should receive information to ensure its clarity and usefulness for the local end user;
> - comply with official language requirements in all media communications;
> - recognize the communication needs of special populations, including populations with low literacy levels and those with perceptual, linguistic or physical challenges;
> - design, deliver and ensure availability of more traditional or alternative forms of communication to meet the needs of special populations;
> - apply citizen engagement, public participation and public consultation techniques to foster feedback from local populations; and
> - take appropriate steps to enhance access to, awareness of, and use of communication materials by diverse populations.
>
> *These guidelines should be adapted to meet local needs*

# ANNEX 2. WHO OUTBREAK COMMUNICATION GUIDELINES[1]

> **WHO/CDS/2005.28**
>
> © World Health Organization 2005
> All rights reserved.
>
> The designations employed and the presentation of the material in this publication do not imply the expression of any opinion whatsoever on the part of the World Health Organization concerning the legal status of any country, territory, city or area or of its authorities, or concerning the delimitation of its frontiers or boundaries. Dotted lines on maps represent approximate border lines for which there may not yet be full agreement.
>
> The mention of specific companies or of certain manufacturers' products does not imply that they are endorsed or recommended by the World Health Organization in preference to others of a similar nature that are not mentioned. Errors and omissions excepted, the names of proprietary products are distinguished by initial capital letters.
>
> All reasonable precautions have been taken by WHO to verify the information contained in this publication. However, the published material is being distributed without warranty of any kind, either express or implied. The responsibility for the interpretation and use of the material lies with the reader. In no event shall the World Health Organization be liable for damages arising from its use.

## I. Background

Disease outbreaks are inevitable, and often unpredictable, events. The environment surrounding an outbreak is unique in all of public health. Outbreaks are frequently marked by uncertainty, confusion and a sense of urgency. Communication, generally through the media, is another feature of the outbreak environment. Unfortunately, examples abound of communication failures which have delayed outbreak control, undermined public trust and compliance, and unnecessarily prolonged economic, social and political turmoil. The World Health Organization (WHO) believes it is now time to acknowledge that communication expertise has become as essential to outbreak control as epidemiological training and laboratory analysis. But what are the best practices for communicating with the public, often through the mass media, during an outbreak?

## II. Guidelines for communicating with the public during outbreaks

In early 2004, WHO began an effort to construct evidence-based, field-tested communication guidance that would promote the public health goal of rapid outbreak control with the least possible disruption to society. The first step in this process was an extensive review of the risk communication literature. During this process, WHO identified risk communication components which had direct relevance to outbreaks. Then, this body of material was distilled into a handful of features strongly associated with communication effectiveness or, when lacking, strongly associated with failures. Finally, these few features were assessed by outbreak control experts from a wide variety of cultures, political systems and economic development. The result of this extensive review, filtered through a broad practical assessment, is a shortlist of outbreak communication best practices. They are listed below.

## 1. Trust

The overriding goal for outbreak communication is to communicate with the public in ways that build, maintain or restore trust. This is true across cultures, political systems and level of country development.

**a.** The consequences of losing the public's trust can be severe in health, economic and political terms. Abundant research and prominent public health examples support the hypothesis that the less people trust those who are supposed to protect them, the more afraid the public will be and less likely they will be to conform their choices and behaviour with outbreak management instructions.

**b.** Senior management must endorse this goal but winning their support for specific trust-building measures faces many practical barriers.

> **I.** This is because these trust-building measures are often counter-intuitive (such as acknowledging uncertainty or avoiding excessive reassurance).
> 
> **II.** Consequently, building trust internally between communicators and policy-makers is critical. Trust is also essential between communicators and technical outbreak response staff who may not see the need of communicating with the public especially if it means diverting them from other tasks. This internal relationship – between communicators, technical staff and policy-makers – is sometimes known as the "trust triangle".
> - It is important that the trust triangle be established before it is needed. This can be complicated because different stakeholders, perhaps represented by different ministries, may have conflicts of interest which will require consensus building among partners.

**c.** Trust in communicating with the public is critical in both directions. Evidence shows that public panic is rare and most rare when people have been candidly informed. But the extent to which outbreak managers trust the public's ability to tolerate incomplete and sometimes alarming information influences communication decision-making and effectiveness.

**d.** Mechanisms of accountability, involvement and transparency are important to establish and maintain trust, and they are especially important to slowly rebuild trust when it is low. Allowing high-profile critics to watch decision-making and even participate, for example, reduces the need for trust and increases trust.

## 2. Announcing early

The parameters of trust are established in the outbreak's first official announcement. This message's timing, candour and comprehensiveness may make it the most important of all outbreak communications.

**a.** In today's globalized, wired world, information about outbreaks is almost impossible to keep hidden from the public. Eventually, the outbreak will be revealed. Therefore, to prevent rumours and misinformation and to frame the event, it is best to announce as early as possible.

**b.** People are more likely to overestimate the risk if information is withheld. And evidence shows that the longer officials withhold worrisome information, the more frightening the information will seem when it is revealed, especially if it is revealed by an outside source.

---

1 We gratefully acknowledge the financial support of the governments of Canada and Japan and the financial and organizational support of the government of Singapore to the WHO Expert Consultation on Outbreak Communications held in Singapore on 21–23 September 2004 and in the production of these guidelines. The issues presented in the guidelines arose from topics raised and discussed at the consultation.

**c.** An announcement must be made when public behaviour might reduce risk or contribute to the containment of the outbreak.

**d.** The small size of an outbreak alone or a lack of information are insufficient arguments to delay an announcement. There are times when even one case, such as an Ebola report, can justify early announcements.

**e.** But there are potential problems.

> **I.** Rapid announcements may surprise important partners who might disagree with the initial assessment. This can be minimized by having well-established communication pathways in place among key and predictable stakeholders. These systems should be tested during routine exchanges or through desktop exercises.
>
> **II.** Early announcements are often based on incomplete and sometimes erroneous information. It is critical to publicly acknowledge that early information may change as further information is developed or verified.

The benefits of early warning outweigh the risks, and even those risks (such as providing inaccurate information) can be minimized with appropriate outbreak communication messages.

## 3. Transparency

Maintaining the public's trust throughout an outbreak requires transparency (i.e. communication that is candid, easily understood, complete and factually accurate). Transparency characterizes the relationship between the outbreak managers and the public. It allows the public to "view" the information-gathering, risk-assessing and decision-making processes associated with outbreak control.

**a.** Transparency provides many benefits, including demonstrating how even at a time of uncertainty and confronting unknowns, outbreak managers are systematically seeking answers.

**b.** Since transparency can also expose weaknesses in outbreak management structures and operations, it provides a strong incentive for deliberative and accountable decision-making.

**c.** Total candour should be the operational goal consistent with generally accepted individual rights, such as patient privacy. The key is to balance the rights of the individual against information directly pertinent to the public good and the public's need and desire for reliable information. Announcing the limits of transparency publicly, and explaining why those limits are being set, is usually well tolerated provided the limits are justified. But if limits to transparency become excuses for unnecessary secretiveness, the likely result will be a loss of public trust.

**d.** Many barriers can block transparency.

> **I.** Economic arguments are often raised, but public health officials' first concern has to be human health. There is, however, an increasing body of evidence showing that recovery from the economic impact of an outbreak is faster when governments have been transparent and have developed a track record of effective outbreak management.
>
> **II.** Media preparation should be an essential component of professional development for public officials. Whenever possible, such preparation should precede each media interaction. It is not a process of preparation of delivery skills so much as preparation of specific messages and answers to likely questions.
>
> **III.** Spokespersons or public officials may not feel confident in delivering bad news or discussing uncertainty.

**IV.** And there might be a fear of revealing weaknesses in infrastructure. Pride, embarrassment, and fear of being blamed can also lead to lack of candour.

**V.** Although these factors are very difficult to manage in an acute situation, culture change among decision-makers and senior technical officers
leading to greater transparency should be one of the strategies in preparedness planning for outbreaks.

Transparency, by itself, cannot ensure trust. The public must see that competent decisions are being made. But in general, greater transparency results in greater trust.

## 4. The public

Understanding the public is critical to effective communication. It is usually difficult to change pre-existing beliefs unless those beliefs are explicitly addressed. And it is nearly impossible to design successful messages that bridge the gap between the expert and the public without knowing what the public thinks.

**a.** Early risk communication was directed at informing the public about technical decisions (known as the "decide and tell" strategy). Today, risk communicators teach that crisis communication is a dialogue.

**b.** It is the job of the communicator to understand the public's beliefs, opinions and knowledge about specific risks. This task is sometimes called "communications surveillance".

**c.** If possible, representatives of the public should be brought into the decision-making process. Often this is not possible, so it becomes the job of the outbreak communication manager to understand and represent those views as decision-making evolves.

**d.** The public's concerns must be appreciated even if they seem unfounded. When a publicly held view has validity, policy-making should be consistent with that view. When a publicly held view is mistaken, it should still be acknowledged publicly and corrected, not ignored, patronized or ridiculed.

**e.** Risk communication messages should include information about what the public can do to make themselves safer. This affords people a sense of control over their own health and safety, which in turn allows them to react to the risk with more reasoned responses.

The public is entitled to information that affects their health and the health of their families. Learning who they are and what they think is critical to successful outbreak communication. Communication about personal preventive measures is particularly useful as it empowers the public to take some responsibility for their own health.

## 5. Planning

The decisions and actions of public health officials have more effect on trust and public risk perception than communication. There is risk communication impact in everything outbreak control managers do, not just in what is said. Therefore, risk communication is most effective when it is integrated with risk analysis and risk management. Risk communication should be incorporated into preparedness planning for major events and in all aspects of an outbreak response.

a. Have a risk communication plan ready before it is needed. Outbreak communication planning must be a part of outbreak management planning from the start. To be effective, outbreak communication cannot be a last-minute, add-on feature to announce decisions.

b. Communication planning is usually led by agency communicators and often ignored by senior management. Because outbreak communication principles include some counter-intuitive notions about dealing with the public, it is a potential hazard to wait for a crisis to tell managers about the need to acknowledge uncertainty or empathize with the public's beliefs and fears.

c. Issues of first announcements, limits of transparency, and other communication components should be agreed upon by senior management and ideally by the political leadership before the crisis is breaking. Central features include answering questions such as: What needs to be done? Who needs to know? Who is the spokesperson? What agency has the lead? And who needs to act? These steps are also placed in context, so they are linked to other ministries and, if need be, the international community.

This does not mean that outbreak communication which has not been planned is doomed to failure. Trust, for example, can develop during an outbreak. But it is far easier to build trust before it is needed.

## III. Conclusion

If implemented effectively, these guidelines for outbreak communication will result in greater public resilience and guide appropriate public participation to support the rapid containment of an outbreak, thus limiting morbidity and mortality. In addition, effective outbreak communication will minimize the damage to a nation's international standing, its economy and its public health infrastructure.

WHO is now extending its outbreak communication activities. Among the next steps is the development of training for communications staff so that they can provide support to WHO country offices during high-profile outbreaks. WHO also plans to assist Member States in building capacity in outbreak communication when requested.

The overriding public health goal is to bring the outbreak under control as quickly as possible, with as little social disruption as possible. Effective outbreak communication is one tool to achieve that goal.

# ANNEX 3. PRINCIPLES AND TECHNIQUES OF EFFECTIVE MEDIA COMMUNICATION

Listed below is a brief summary of the principles and techniques of effective media communication. This summary is based upon a review of the scientific and practitioner literature. These principles and techniques are covered in the seven steps. They are repeated and summarized here for the convenience of the reader. More information on each principle and technique can be found in earlier sections of this handbook.

## I. Principles and techniques

### 1. Accept the media as a legitimate partner

- Recognize that effective media communication in an emergency or crisis:
  - enables the media to play a constructive role in protecting the public's health;
  - enables public health officials to reach a wide range of stakeholders; and
  - enables public health officials, in cooperation with the media, to build trust, calm a nervous public, provide needed information, encourage cooperative behaviours, and save lives.
- Demonstrate respect for the media by keeping them well informed of decisions and actions.
- Establish good working relationships with media contacts before an emergency arises.
- Include journalists in public emergency response planning exercises.
- Be polite and courteous at all times, even if the reporter is not.
- Avoid embarrassing reporters.
- Provide information for on-site reporters on the location of electrical outlets, public telephones, rest rooms, hotels, restaurants and other amenities.
- Avoid being defensive or argumentative during interviews.
- Include elements in interviews that make a story interesting to the media, including examples, stories and other aspects that influence public perceptions of risk, concern and outrage.
- Use a wide range of media communication channels to engage and involve people.
- Adhere to the highest ethical standards – recognize that people hold you professionally and ethically accountable.
- Strive to inform editors and reporters of agency preparedness for a public health emergency.
- Offer to follow-up on questions that cannot be addressed immediately.
- Strive for "win-win" media outcomes.
- Involve the media in training exercises and preparedness drills.

### 2. Plan thoroughly and carefully for all media interactions

- Assess the cultural diversity and socioeconomic level of the target populations.
- Assess internal media-relations capabilities.
- Recognize that all communication activities and materials should reflect the diverse nature of societies in a fair, representative and inclusive manner.

- Begin all communication planning efforts with clear and explicit goals – such as:
  - informing and educating;
  - improving knowledge and understanding;
  - building, maintaining or restoring trust;
  - guiding and encouraging appropriate attitudes, decisions, actions and behaviours; and
  - encouraging dialogue, collaboration and cooperation.
- Develop a written communication plan.
- Develop a partner communication strategy.
- Establish coordination in situations involving multiple agencies.
- Identify important stakeholders and subgroups within the audience as targets for your messages.
- Prepare a limited number of key messages in advance of potential public health emergencies.
- Post the key messages and supporting information on your own well-publicized web site.
- Pre-test messages before using them during an interview.
- Respect diversity and multiculturalism while developing messages.
- Train key personnel – including technical staff – in basic, intermediate and advanced media communication skills.
- Practise media communication skills regularly.
- Never say anything "off-the-record" that you would not want to see quoted and attributed to you.
- Recruit media spokespersons who have effective presentation and personal interaction skills.
- Provide training for high-ranking government officials who play a major role in communication with the media.
- Provide well-developed talking points for those who play a leading role in communication with the media.
- Recognize and reward spokespersons who are successful in getting their key messages included in media stories.
- Anticipate questions and issues that might be raised during an interview.
- Train spokespersons in how to redirect an interview (or get it back on track) using bridging phrases such as "what is really important to know is…".
- Agree with the reporter in advance on logistics and topic – for example, the length, location, and specific topic of the interview – but realize that the reporter may attempt to stray from the agreed topic.
- Make needed changes in strategy and messages based on monitoring activities, evaluation efforts and feedback.
- Work proactively to frame stories rather than waiting until others have defined the story and then reacting.
- Carefully evaluate media communication efforts and learn from mistakes.
- Share with others what you have learned from working with the media.

### 3. Meet the functional needs of the media

- Assess the needs of the media.
- Be accessible to reporters.
- Respect their deadlines.
- Accept that news reports will simplify and abbreviate your messages.
- Devise a schedule to brief the media regularly during an emergency, even if updates are not "newsworthy" by their standards – open and regular communication helps to build trust and fill information voids.

- Refer journalists to your web site for further information.
- Share a limited number of key messages for media interviews.
- Repeat your key messages several times during news conferences and media interviews.
- Provide accurate, appropriate and useful information tailored to the needs of each type of media, such as sound bites, background videotape, and other visual materials for television.
- Provide background material for reporters on basic and complex issues on your web site and as part of media information packets and kits.
- Be careful when providing numbers to reporters – these can easily be misinterpreted or misunderstood.
- Stick to the agreed topic during the interview – do not digress.
- If you do not know the answer to a question, focus on what you do know, tell the reporter what actions you will take to get an answer, and follow up in a timely manner.
- If asked for information that is the responsibility of another individual or organization, refer the reporter to that individual or organization.
- Offer reporters the opportunity to do follow-up interviews with subject-matter experts.
- Strive for brevity, but respect the reporter's desire for information.
- Hold media availability sessions where partners in the response effort are available for questioning in one place at one time.
- Remember that it benefits the reporter and the agency when a story is accurate.
- Before an emergency occurs, meet with editors and with reporters who would cover the story.
- Work to establish durable relationships with reporters and editors.
- Promise only that which can be delivered, then follow through.

## 4. Be candid and open with reporters

- Be first to share bad news about an issue or your organization, but be sure to put it into context.
- If the answer to a question is unknown or uncertain, and if the reporter is not reporting in real time, express a willingness to get back to the reporter with a response by an agreed deadline.
- Be first and proactive in disclosing information about an emergency, emphasizing appropriate reservations about data and information reliability.
- Recognize that most journalists maintain a "healthy scepticism" of sources, and trust by the media is earned – do not ask to be trusted.
- Ask the reporter to restate a question if you do not understand it.
- Hold frequent media events to fill information voids.
- Do not minimize or exaggerate the level of risk.
- Acknowledge uncertainty.
- Be careful about comparing the risk of one event to another.
- Do not offer unreasonable reassurances (i.e. unwarranted by the available information).
- Make corrections quickly if errors are made or if the facts change.
- Discuss data and information uncertainties, strengths and weaknesses – including those identified by other credible sources.
- Cite ranges of risk estimates when appropriate.
- Support your messages with case studies and data.
- If credible authorities disagree on the best course of action, be prepared to disclose the rationale for those disagreements, and why your agency has decided to take one particular course of action over another.
- Be especially careful when asked to speculate or answer extreme or baseless "what if" questions, especially on worst-case scenarios.
- Avoid speaking in absolutes.
- Tell the truth.

## 5. Listen to the target audience

- Do not make assumptions about what viewers, listeners and readers know, think or want done about risks.
- If time and resources allow, prior to a media interview, review the available data and information on public perceptions, attitudes, opinions, beliefs and likely responses regarding an event or risk. Such information may have been obtained through interviews, facilitated discussion groups, information exchanges, expert availability sessions, public hearings, advisory group meetings, hotline call-in logs, and surveys.
- Monitor and analyse information about the event appearing in media outlets, including the internet.
- Identify with the target audience of the media interview, and present information in a format that aids understanding and helps people to act accordingly.
- During interviews and news conferences, acknowledge the validity of people's emotions and fears.
- Be empathetic.
- Target media channels that encourage listening, feedback, participation and dialogue.
- Recognize that competing agendas, symbolic meanings, and broader social, cultural, economic or political considerations often complicate the task of effective media communication.
- Recognize that although public health officials may speak in terms of controlling "morbidity and mortality" rates, more important issues for some audiences may be whether people are being treated fairly in terms of access to care and medical resources.

## 6. Coordinate, collaborate and act in partnership with other credible sources

- Develop procedures for coordinating the activities of media spokespersons from multiple agencies and organizations.
- Establish links to the web sites of partner organizations.
- Recognize that every organization has its own culture and this culture impacts upon how and what it tries to communicate.
- To the extent possible, act in partnership with other organizations in preparing messages in advance of potential emergencies.
- Share and coordinate messages with partner organizations prior to media interviews or news conferences.
- Encourage partner organizations to repeat or echo the same key messages – such repetition and echoing by many voices helps to reinforce the key messages for target audiences.
- In situations involving multiple agencies, determine information clearance and approval procedures in advance when possible.
- Aim for consistency of key messages across agencies – if real differences in opinion do exist be inclined to disclose the areas of disagreement and explain why your agency is choosing one course of action over another.
- Develop a contingency plan for when partners cannot engage in consistent messaging – be prepared to make an extra effort to listen to their concerns, understand their point of view, negotiate differences, and apply pressure if required and appropriate.
- Devote effort and resources to building bridges, partnerships and alliances with other organizations (including potential or established critics) before an emergency occurs.
- Consult with internal and external partners to determine which organization should take the lead in responding to media enquiries, and document the agreements reached.
- Discuss ownership of specific topics or issues in advance to avoid one partner treading upon the perceived territory of another.

- Identify credible and authoritative sources of information that can be used to support messages in potential emergencies.
- Develop a plan for using information from other organizations in potential emergencies.
- Develop contact lists of external subject-matter experts able and willing to speak to the media on issues associated with potential emergencies.
- Cite as part of your message credible and authoritative sources that believe what you believe.
- Issue media communications together with, or through, individuals or organizations believed to be credible and trustworthy by the target audience.

## 7. Speak clearly and with compassion

- Be aware that people want to know that you care before they care what you know.
- Use clear, non-technical language.
- Explain medical or technical terms in clear language when they are used.
- Use graphics or other pictorial material to clarify and strengthen messages.
- Respect the unique information needs of special and diverse audiences.
- Express genuine empathy when responding to questions about loss – acknowledge the tragedy of illness, injury or death.
- Personalize risk data by using stories, narratives, examples and anecdotes that make technical data easier to understand.
- Avoid distant, abstract and unfeeling language about harm, deaths, injuries and illnesses.
- Acknowledge and respond (in words, gestures and actions) to the emotions people express, such as anxiety, fear, worry, anger, outrage and helplessness.
- Acknowledge and respond to the distinctions people view as important in evaluating risks, such as perceived benefits, control, fairness, dread, whether the risk is natural or man-made, and effects on children.
- Be careful to use risk comparisons only to help put risks in perspective and context, and not to suggest that one risk is like another – avoid comparisons that trivialize the problem, that attempt to minimize anxiety, or that appear to be trying to settle the question of whether a risk is acceptable.
- Give people a sense of control by identifying specific actions they can take to protect themselves.
- Identify significant misinformation, being aware that repeating it may give it unwanted attention.
- Recognize that saying "no comment" without explanation or qualification is often perceived as guilt or hiding something – consider saying instead "I wish I could answer that. However…".
- Be sensitive to local norms, such as those relating to speech and dress.
- Always try to include in a media interview a discussion of actions under way by the agency, or actions that can be taken by the public.

# ANNEX 4. SAMPLE MEDIA COMMUNICATION PLAN CONTENTS

The following "Table of Contents" is only an example and should be adapted to meet local needs.

## I. Signed endorsement from the agency director

## II. Policies

| |
|---|
| Goals |
| Responsibilities |
| Emergency notification |
| Activation of the media communication plan |
| Information verification and approval |
| Disclosure of sensitive information |
| Designated spokespersons |
| Communication roles and responsibilities |
| Creating a multi-agency Joint Information Centre |
| Web site updates |

## III. Procedures, rosters and checklists

| |
|---|
| Emergency notification protocol |
| Emergency response list |
| Media contact sheet |
| External emergency notification roster |
| Agency spokespersons |
| Subject matter experts |
| Communication checklist |
| Communication team roles and responsibilities |
| Communication team/function master assignment checklist |
| Communication team individual assignment sheets |
| Emergency communication event assessment |
| Key messages |
| Location and inventory of fact sheets, media kits, and other informational materials |

# ANNEX 5. SAMPLE LETTER OF ENDORSEMENT[1] BY THE AGENCY DIRECTOR OF THE MEDIA COMMUNICATION PLAN

<agency name>                <agency logo>

<telephone>                                                      <addressee>

<fax>

<email>

<reference>

                                                                  <date>

<salutation>

Communication is a key factor in the response of the agency to any emergency. When a public health emergency arises, timely, accurate, clear, concise and credible messages have a tremendous impact on how the public reacts during an event, and on its perception of public health.

The agency's media emergency communication plan has been designed as a blueprint to aid the agency in responding to an intentional, unintentional or naturally occurring event that creates a public health threat. It spells out the crucial first steps and formalizes our policies.

The goals of this media emergency communication plan are to:

- rapidly provide access to timely, accurate, clear, consistent and credible information to the public, the media, emergency responders, health care providers, policy-makers and other interested parties;
- address, as quickly as possible, rumours, inaccuracies and misperceptions;
- coordinate communication efforts with partner organizations;
- fulfil information requests from the media, public, staff and other interested or affected parties;
- eliminate or reduce public fear or inappropriate behaviour; and
- direct public action.

I have reviewed and approved the attached media emergency communication plan. I hereby pronounce that this is the plan to follow in a public health emergency.

                         <closing>

                         <signature block>

                         <name and title of agency director>

---

1  To be published as part of the agency's written media communication plan.

# ANNEX 6. QUESTIONS FREQUENTLY ASKED BY JOURNALISTS AND THE PUBLIC DURING DISEASE OUTBREAKS

The following questions have often been asked by journalists and the public during past disease outbreaks. Such questions could be further refined by grouping them according to themes, such as clinical traits, epidemiological traits, accountability, blame, vulnerable groups and protective actions.

| |
|---|
| How contagious is the disease? |
| Can people be vaccinated? Will antibiotics and antiviral medicines work? How effective are vaccinations, antibiotics or antiviral medicines for those with the disease? How effective are vaccinations, antibiotics, or antiviral medicines for those who do not have the disease? How fast do the vaccines or antibiotics work? |
| What are the signs and symptoms of the disease? |
| Who is in charge of the disease control effort? How are you coordinating the efforts among responsible agencies? |
| Is the outbreak due to terrorism? Has the disease been "weaponized"? How certain are you that it is not a deliberate release? What if the disease is a genetically altered strain that is resistant to any known medical treatment? |
| What makes you think the disease control strategies of the past will work today? |
| What is being done to stop the spread of the disease? |
| What kind of medical care is available to the population at risk? Are there enough medical care facilities? What happens if these care facilities are overwhelmed by demand? |
| What resources are being used to respond to the disease outbreak? |
| Can the disease be treated? How effective is treatment? Are there strains of the disease that cannot be treated? |
| How does one know if the vaccinations, antibiotics or antiviral medicines are working? |
| Are laboratories able to quickly diagnose the disease? How long does confirmation take? |
| Is the disease airborne? Waterborne? |
| Can people get the disease from insects, pets, farm animals and wild animals? |
| What are the authorities in areas not affected doing to prepare for an outbreak? |
| How are the vaccines made? How are the antibiotics and antiviral medicines made? Are there enough vaccines, antibiotics or antiviral medicines for everyone who wants them? Who will pay for vaccines, antibiotics or antiviral medicines? |
| How will vaccines, antibiotics and antiviral medicines be distributed? How much time will be needed? Where can people be vaccinated, get antibiotics or get antiviral medicines? If there is a shortage, who will get priority? Who will make these decisions? |

# ANNEXES

| |
|---|
| What should people do if they think they have the disease? |
| Do you recommend that people get vaccinated, take antibiotics or take antiviral medicines now? How long does protection last? |
| Are the vaccines, antibiotics or antiviral medicines licensed and approved? What is the expiration date? Should people be concerned? |
| Are the vaccines, antibiotics or antiviral medicines safe? How do you know? What studies have been done to demonstrate their safety? |
| Who should not get vaccinated, should not take antibiotics, or should not take antiviral medicines? What can these people do to protect themselves? |
| Who will tell people when to be vaccinated, take antibiotics, or take antiviral medicines? |
| Is there an adequate supply of medicines available to treat the complications of vaccination, or of taking antibiotics or antiviral medicines? |
| What are the alternatives to vaccination, antibiotics, or antiviral medicines? |
| How safe are people who get vaccinated, take antibiotics or take antiviral medicines? |
| Do you have a contingency plan if current control measures fail? |
| What does the contingency plan say? What is the worst case? |
| Who developed and approved the plan? |
| What is the risk to the population? How many could die? |
| How prepared were you for the disease outbreak? |
| How do you know whether the outbreak is real? Could it be a false alarm? |
| If people get sick from the vaccination, from taking antibiotics or from taking antiviral medicines, who will care for their families, pets, homes and property? |
| How common are side-effects from vaccination, taking antibiotics or taking antiviral medicines? What are the risks of each side-effect occurring? |
| Can pets and farm animals be vaccinated, or be given antibiotics or antiviral medicines? |
| Can people with HIV/AIDS, transplants, cancer and other causes of weakened immune systems be treated? |
| Can elderly people and children be treated? Can pregnant women be treated? |
| What are you recommending for your own family? |
| How long does it take for the vaccination, antibiotics or antiviral medicines to protect people against the disease? |
| Are there people who will not be protected even after getting vaccinated, taking antibiotics or taking antiviral medicines? How many people are in this category? What are their options? |
| How can people prevent the disease from spreading to others? |
| Will people be forced to be vaccinated, take antibiotics or take antiviral medicines? |
| Will infected people be isolated or quarantined? |
| How long will quarantine and isolation last? |

| |
|---|
| What is the legal basis for quarantine and isolation? |
| How effective is quarantine and isolation in preventing the spread of the disease? |
| How will bills be paid while people are in quarantine or isolation? |
| How will people get health care, water, food and other services while in quarantine or isolation? |
| Where will people in quarantine or isolation be placed? |
| Will people in quarantine or isolation be isolated from each other? |
| Under what circumstances will people be put in quarantine or isolation? |
| What are the legal rights of a person who is quarantined or isolated? |
| Are there alternatives to quarantine and isolation? |
| How is quarantine or isolation done? |
| What is life like in quarantine or isolation? |
| Under what circumstances would a large-scale quarantine or isolation effort be started? |
| If someone becomes sick in quarantine or isolation, who will care for them? How good will the medical care be? |
| Will people in quarantine or isolation be able to communicate with family and friends? |
| Will a person's job be protected while they are in quarantine or isolation? |
| What will happen to people who refuse to be quarantined or isolated? |
| Can people get sick when in quarantine or isolation? |
| What happens if someone dies in quarantine or isolation? |
| What happens to facilities after they are used for quarantine or isolation? |
| Can people bring their pets/family/friends into a quarantine or isolation facility? |
| Can a community refuse to have a quarantine or isolation facility located nearby? |
| How will quarantine and isolation affect community life, including transportation? |
| Are there differences of opinion among experts about the need for and effectiveness of quarantine or isolation procedures? |
| After release from quarantine or isolation, will people be able to go back to work? |
| What are the personal, family and job consequences for people in quarantine or isolation? |
| In quarantine or isolation, will special provisions be made for cultural, religious and ethnic beliefs and values? |
| Who will pay the costs for quarantine or isolation? |
| Who will pay the costs for lost wages of people in quarantine or isolation? |

# ANNEX 7. EFFECTIVELY COMMUNICATING RISK NUMBERS

There are many ways to express numerical risk information, and each expression communicates different information. It is therefore important to understand the various ways in which risk can be expressed and the different meanings and implications of each approach. The types of measures that can be used to communicate risk include:

- concentrations – such as parts per million or per billion;
- probabilities – i.e. the likelihood of an event; and
- quantities – such as how many anthrax spores were in a letter.

## I. Factors that influence effective risk number communication

When communicating risk information it is important to be aware of the following factors.

### 1. Framing

Responses to information about risk are highly dependent upon how the information is framed. For example, presenting risk information in terms of "lives lost" versus "lives saved" can have a profound affect on how people respond. In one study, doctors were presented with a hypothetical choice between two cancer therapies with different probabilities of success and failure. Half were told about the relative chances of dying while the rest had the same information presented in terms of survival rates. This change in framing – even though the results were the same – more than doubled the number of doctors choosing one alternative. Because of framing effects, and because outcomes can be measured against different reference points (as with the bottle half-full or half-empty), no risk number will ever be the "right number". Each way of expressing a risk "frames" it differently and thus will have a different impact on the audience.

### 2. Units

Risk is often expressed as the expected number of deaths (or other measure) per unit of x per duration of exposure y. The ways of expressing this number, however, are not equivalent and different measures will often strike an audience as being more or less appropriate, frightening or comprehensible. For example, one measure commonly used to express numerical risk is lost life expectancy. However, this measure gives more weight to early deaths and less to deaths in old age. Risk is also frequently expressed in terms of lost workdays. However, this measure gives virtually no weight to the lives of children, non-working people, and retired people.

### 3. Absolute vs relative risk

Responses to risk messages – especially when communicating increases or decreases in risk – depend critically upon whether the probabilities are presented in absolute terms ("the probability was 2% and is now 4%") or relative terms (as in "the probability has doubled" or "this group suffers twice the normal risk of…"). The latter approach can be seriously misleading. Information about relative risk can result in misperceptions if information about the baseline probabilities is not made clear.

## 4. Scale

Transformations of scale can radically change perceptions of risk numbers. For example, in communicating concentrations, the expression "six parts per billion" sounds a great deal larger than 0.006 parts per million, even though they are the same. Scale is also a factor in communicating probabilities. For example, a risk agent expected to result in the death of 1.4 people in every 1000 can equally be expressed as:

- "the risk is 0.0014";
- "the risk is 0.14%"; or
- in a community of a thousand people, we could expect 1.4 to die as a result of exposure.

Although these alternatives are equivalent, their meanings to audiences (and hence their effect) may not be identical. The first term may make the risk seem smaller, while the last term may make it seem larger. Confusion can often be avoided by embedding risk numbers in words that help clarify their meaning. For example, "a risk of 0.047" is comprehensible to only a few people. By comparison, it is much easier to understand that about 5 people in an auditorium of 100 would be affected. This embedding process can also be accomplished through visuals, including graphs, charts, animation and pictures.

## 5. Other adverse effects

Risk numbers that focus only on death may tell only one part of the story. Other possible adverse health consequences of interest may include birth defects, mutations and genetic damage, immune-system damage, neurological damage, organ damage, fertility problems and behavioural disorders.

## 6. Estimates

Many risk numbers are estimates based on modelling. Because they are based on models, risk estimates produced by risk assessments (instead of counting) often have substantial margins of error. In some cases, uncertainties in risk estimates arise from the use of different assumptions and extrapolations. In other cases, uncertainties arise because the risk is very low and measurement is very difficult. Because of uncertainties, one approach to communicating risk numbers is to report the most likely estimate of risk. A second approach is to report the upper boundary, "worst case" or maximum estimate of risk. A third approach is to report the most likely estimate, along with the highest and lowest estimates from credible sources. For example, "Our best estimate is a and our cautious worst-case estimate is b with the highest estimate we have heard, from scientists at University X, is c".

## 7. Over-simplification

A common tendency in attempting to clarify risk numbers is to oversimplify. Clarity is not, however, the same thing as oversimplification. Most people, if sufficiently motivated, are capable of understanding quite complex quantitative information.

## 8. Context

In presenting risk numbers, it is often useful to explain how they were obtained. Demystifying the risk-assessment process has several benefits. Perhaps most importantly, it enables the presenter to make points that may be important for people to understand. For example, it allows the point to be made that the presence of a risk agent does not necessarily signify a significant health risk. It is often extremely difficult to communicate that for a risk agent to pose a threat, an exposure route to people or the things they value has to be in place. Explaining the risk assessment process also allows the presenter to make a second critical point. Even after an exposure route is established, the next important question is the concentration of the risk agent that may reach people. Concentration amounts are typically far lower than the concentration amounts at the source. Moreover, they often become even lower with the passage of time and distance. Risk assessors consider not only whether a risk agent is present but also how much is present.

## 9. Biases

The most common expression of risk is in terms of probabilities. Probabilities obey well-known mathematical laws. However the brain tends to manipulate or simplify probabilities in ways that contravene these laws. These manipulations often lead to various biases in dealing with probabilities. Some of the most relevant are:

- **availability bias** – events are perceived to be more frequent if examples are easily brought to mind, with memorable events therefore seeming more common;
- **confirmation bias** – once a view has been formed, new evidence is generally made to fit, contrary information is filtered out, ambiguous data interpreted as confirmation, and consistent information seen as "proof"; and
- **overconfidence** – we think our predictions or estimates are more likely to be correct than they really are, and this bias appears to affect almost all professions.

# II. Comparisons

Risk numbers are often communicated as part of a comparison. The goal of comparisons is to make the original risk number more meaningful by comparing it to other numbers. For example, small probabilities are often difficult to conceptualize (just how small is "1 in 10 million" or "a probability of 0.00015"?). Although risk comparisons can provide a yardstick and are therefore useful for putting numbers in perspective, they can also create their own problems. For example, use of the concentration comparisons found in **TABLE ONE** can lead to disagreements. The statement "one part per million of a contaminant is equal to one drop in an Olympic-size swimming pool" or "one drop of vermouth in a million-gallon martini" is typically intended to help the reader understand how "small" an amount is. However, for some individuals, such comparisons appear to trivialize the problem and to prejudge their acceptability. Furthermore, concentration comparisons can sometimes be misleading since risk agents vary widely in potency – one drop of some biological agents in a community reservoir can kill many people, while one drop of other biological agents will have no effect whatsoever. Comparing the probabilities associated with different risks has many of the same problems. For example, it is often tempting to use the numbers found in **TABLE TWO** to make the following type of argument:

- "The risk of *a* (contracting smallpox or SARS) is lower than the risk of *b* (injured or killed while driving a car). Since you (the target audience) find *b* acceptable, you are obliged to find *a* acceptable."

This argument appears to have a basic flaw in its logic and trying to use it could severely damage trust and credibility. Some receivers of the comparison will analyse the argument this way:

- "I do not have to accept the (small) added risk of contracting smallpox or SARS just because I accept the (perhaps larger, but voluntary and personally beneficial) risk of driving my car. In deciding about the acceptability of risks, I consider many factors, only one of them being the size of the risk; and I prefer to do my own evaluation."

Probabilities are only one of many kinds of information upon which people base decisions about risk acceptability. Risk numbers cannot pre-empt those decisions. Explanations of risk numbers are unlikely to be successful if the explanation appears to be trying to settle the question of whether a risk is acceptable.

More research is needed to clarify which comparisons are most effective and why. Many variables affect their success, including context and the trustworthiness of the source of the comparison. With this caution in mind, the most effective comparisons appear to be:

- comparisons of the same risk at two different times;
- comparisons with a regulatory standard;
- comparisons with different estimates of the same risk;
- comparisons of the risk of doing something versus not doing it;
- comparisons of alternative solutions to the same problem; and
- comparisons with the same risk as experienced in other places.

All these types of comparisons have some claim to relevance and legitimacy.

The most difficult comparisons to communicate effectively are those that disregard the risk perception factors people consider important in evaluating risks. The most important of these include trustworthiness, fairness, benefits, alternatives, control, dread, catastrophic potential and familiarity. For example, the entries in **TABLE TWO** juxtapose voluntary and involuntary risks and widely different forms of death (accident, cancer). Furthermore, the numbers in such tables are often estimates and can give a false impression of precision.

### TABLE ONE: Concentration comparisons[1]

| Unit | 1 part per million | 1 part per billion | 1 part per trillion |
| --- | --- | --- | --- |
| Length | 1 inch in 16 miles | 1 inch in 16 000 miles | 1 inch in 16 000 000 miles (or a 6-inch leap on a journey to the sun) |
| Time | 1 min. in 2 years | 1 sec. in 32 years | 1 sec. in 320 centuries (or 0.06 sec. since the birth of Jesus Christ) |
| Money | 1 cent in $10 000 | 1 cent in $10 000 000 | 1 cent in $10 000 000 000 |
| Weight | 1 oz. in 31 tons | 1 pinch salt in 10 tons of potato chips | 1 pinch salt in 10 000 tons of potato chips |
| Volume | 1 drop vermouth in 80 "fifths" of gin | 1 drop vermouth in 500 barrels of gin | 1 drop of vermouth in a pool of gin covering the area of a football field 43 ft. deep |
| Area | 1 square foot in 23 acres | 1 square inch in a 160-acre farm | 1 square foot in the state of Indiana (or 1 large grain of sand on the surface of Daytona Beach) |
| Action | 1 lob in 1200 tennis matches | 1 lob in 1200 000 tennis matches | 1 lob in 1 200 000 000 tennis matches |
| Quality | 1 bad apple in 2000 barrels | 1 bad apple in 2 000 000 barrels | 1 bad apple in 2 000 000 000 barrels |

1 Source: Rowe WD et al. (1984) (data based on US metrics)

## TABLE TWO: Various annual and lifetime risks[1]

| Cause of death or harm | Annual risk | Lifetime risk |
|---|---|---|
| Heart disease | 1 in 300 | 1 in 4 |
| Cancer (all forms) | 1 in 510 | 1 in 7 |
| Pneumonia | 1 in 4300 | 1 in 57 |
| Plague | 1 in 19 000 000 | 1 in 240 000 |
| Anthrax (2001) | 1 in 56 000 000 | 1 in 730 000 |
| Suicide | 1 in 9200 | 1 in 120 |
| Criminal homicide | 1 in 18 000 | 1 in 240 |
| Motor vehicle accident | 1 in 6700 | 1 in 88 |
| Commercial aircraft accident | 1 in 3 100 000 | 1 in 40 000 |
| Passenger train accident | 1 in 70 000 000 | 1 in 920 000 |
| Occupational accident | 1 in 48 000 | 1 in 620 |
| Accidental electrocution | 1 in 300 000 | 1 in 4000 |
| Lightning | 1 in 3 000 000 | 1 in 39 000 |
| Shark Attack | 1 in 280 000 000 | 1 in 3 700 000 |

1 Ropeik D, Gray G (2002) (data based on US population)

# III. Quality control

Risk numbers are only as good as the studies from which they are derived. As a result, the following questions should be asked:

## 1. Questions about credibility

- Have the researchers only found a statistical correlation or a difference that has actual health implications?
- Have the findings been published in a peer-reviewed journal?
- Do the researchers have an established track record?
- What are the affiliations of the researcher(s)?
- What is the reputation of these organizations or institutions?

## 2. Questions about methods

- What research methods were used?
- Are these conventional methods?
- Have the results been replicated?
- What do other professionals in the field think about these methods?
- Is the sample size adequate to make a conclusion?
- If this involves a new diagnostic test, is the test validated to truly measure what it claims? How often is the test falsely negative or falsely positive?

## 3. Questions about conclusions

- Have important caveats been prominently included?
- Are the findings preliminary?
- Are there other possible interpretations of the data?
- Do the findings differ markedly from previous studies?
- Are the findings based on small or unrepresentative samples?
- Is the abstract a fair reflection of the report?
- To what extent, if any, can the findings be generalized?

# ANNEX 8. FACTORS IN RISK PERCEPTION

Each of the factors listed below can significantly affect the perception of risk, and each functions against a complex backdrop of social and cultural values.

## I. Summary of risk perception factors

### 1. Voluntariness
Risks from activities considered to be involuntary or imposed (for example, exposure to chemicals and radiation from a terrorist attack using chemical weapons or dirty bombs) are judged to be greater, and are therefore less readily accepted, than risks from voluntary activities (such as smoking, sunbathing or mountain climbing).

### 2. Controllability
Risks from activities considered to be under the control of others (such as the release of nerve gas in a coordinated series of terrorist attacks) are judged to be greater, and are less readily accepted than those from activities considered to be under the control of the individual (such as driving an automobile or riding a bicycle).

### 3. Familiarity
Risks resulting from activities viewed as unfamiliar (such as travel leading to exposure to exotic-sounding infectious diseases) are judged greater than risks resulting from activities viewed as familiar (such as household work).

### 4. Fairness
Risks from activities believed to be unfair or to involve unfair processes (such as inequities in the location of medical facilities) are judged greater than risks from "fair" activities (such as widespread vaccinations).

### 5. Benefits
Risks from activities that seem to have unclear, questionable or diffused personal or economic benefits (for example, proximity to waste-disposal facilities) are judged to be greater than risks resulting from activities with clear benefits (for example, employment or automobile driving).

### 6. Catastrophic potential
Risks from activities associated with potentially high numbers of deaths and injuries grouped in time and space (for example, major terrorist attacks using biological, chemical or nuclear weapons) are judged to be greater than risks from activities that cause deaths and injuries scattered (often apparently randomly) in time and space (for example, household accidents).

### 7. Understanding
Poorly understood risks (such as the health effects of long-term exposure to low doses of toxic chemicals or radiation) are judged to be greater than risks that are well understood or self-explanatory (such as pedestrian accidents or slipping on ice).

### 8. Uncertainty
Risks that are relatively unknown or highly uncertain (such as those associated with genetic engineering) are judged to be greater than risks from activities that appear to be relatively well known to science (such as actuarial risk data related to automobile accidents).

## 9. Effects on children

Activities that appear to put children specifically at risk (such as drinking milk contaminated with radiation or toxic chemicals or pregnant women exposed to radiation or toxic chemicals) are judged to carry greater risks than more-general activities (such as employment).

## 10. Victim identity

Risks from activities that produce identifiable victims (such as an individual worker exposed to high levels of toxic chemicals or radiation, or a child who falls down a well) are judged to be greater than risks from activities that produce statistical victim profiles (such as automobile accidents).

## 11. Dread

Risks from activities that evoke fear, terror or anxiety due to the horrific consequences of exposure (for example to HIV, radiation sickness, cancer, Ebola or smallpox) are judged to be greater than risks from activities that do not arouse such feelings or emotions regarding exposure (for example to common colds or household accidents).

## 12. Trust

Risks from activities associated with individuals, institutions or organizations lacking in trust and credibility (for example, chemical companies or nuclear power plants with poor safety records) are judged to be greater than risks from activities associated with trustworthy and credible sources (for example, regulatory agencies that achieve high levels of compliance from regulated industries).

## 13. Media attention

Risks from activities that generate considerable media attention (such as anthrax attacks using the postal system or accidents at nuclear power plants) are judged to be greater than risks from activities that generate little media attention (such as occupational accidents).

## 14. Accident history

Activities with a history of major accidents or incidents, or frequent minor accidents or incidents (such as leaks from waste-disposal facilities) are judged to carry greater risks than activities with little or no such history (such as recombinant DNA experimentation).

## 15. Reversibility

The risks of potentially irreversible adverse effects (such as birth defects from exposure to a toxic substance or radiation) are judged to be greater than risks considered to be reversible (for example, sports injuries).

## 16. Personal stake

Activities viewed as placing people or their families personally and directly at risk (such as living near a waste-disposal site) are judged to carry greater risks than activities that appear to pose no direct or personal threat (such as the disposal of waste in remote areas).

## 17. Ethical and moral status

Risks from activities believed to be ethically objectionable or morally wrong (such as providing diluted or outdated vaccines for an economically distressed community) are judged to be greater than the risks from ethically neutral activities (such as the side-effects of medication).

## 18. Human versus natural origin

Risks generated by human action, failure or incompetence (such as negligence, inadequate safeguards or operator error) are judged to be greater than risks believed to be caused by nature or "acts of god" (such as exposure to geological radon or cosmic rays).

# ANNEX 9. HOW PEOPLE FORM RISK PERCEPTIONS AND MAKE RISK JUDGEMENTS

Individual perceptions or assessment of risk is typically based on a combination of hazard and risk-perception factors. Risk-perception factors are numerous and are more fully dealt with in **ANNEX 8**. Examples include concepts such as "voluntariness", "fairness", "controllability" and "dread", and are often associated with strong emotional overtones such as outrage, fear and high anxiety. As a result, such factors predispose an individual to react emotionally to risk information which in turn can significantly amplify levels of worry, public anxiety, and negative outcomes. The worries and concerns people have are also determined by their own values, life experiences, intuition, and by social and cultural factors.

In addition to risk-perception factors, people also use a large number of mental short-cuts (called "heuristics" in the communications research literature) to calculate the probability that an adverse action or event will happen. Because of these short-cuts, people may make biased judgements, or use only a small amount of the available information when making decisions about risk. For example, people often assign greater probability to events about which they are frequently reminded (for example, by the news media or scientific literature, or in discussions with friends or colleagues) or to events that are easy to recall or imagine through concrete examples or dramatic images. People consistently overestimate the occurrences of rare and dramatic causes of fatalities while underestimating the frequency of more common causes of death. Deaths from botulism, for example, are estimated to be more common than they actually are, while deaths from diabetes and stroke are estimated to be less frequent than they actually are. All of these processes can attract journalists to write stories, and effective emergency communication must therefore take account of the psychological, social, cultural and physical dimensions of risk.

Research indicates that people's perception of risk is a function of two main sets of risk-perception factors:

- those reflecting the degree to which the risk is ***unknown***; and
- those reflecting the degree to which the risk is ***dreaded***.

Unknown risks include those that are uncertain, not well understood, unobservable, new or have delayed consequences. Dread reflects the degree to which something is perceived to be potentially catastrophic, involuntary, uncontrollable, affecting future generations or unfair. These two factors can be visualized with the degree of dread plotted along the x-axis and the degree to which something is unknown on the y-axis. Placing an event, activity or technology correctly on this graph is highly predictive of the media and public response to it. For example, media coverage and public demands for regulation tend to be greatest for those events, activities or technologies perceived to be the most unknown and dreaded.

As an example, it was learned in the mid-1990s that "mad cow disease" was related to Creutzfeldt-Jakob Disease (CJD) in humans. The disease rated highly in degree of dread – its symptoms were horrific, it was fatal, the risk was largely involuntary (exposure could only be avoided by not eating meat), and the risk was seen as uncontrollable by the individual. It also ranked highly along the unknown axis because the disease was not well understood by scientists, there was no known vaccine or cure and the onset of symptoms was delayed for years. The responses of the media and the public were correspondingly dramatic as predicted by **FIGURE NINE**.

## FIGURE NINE: FACTORS AFFECTING RISK PERCEPTION

**Unknown risk**

unobservable
delayed effect
new
risks unknown to science

Medical x-rays

Outbreaks of exotic disease
e.g., Creutzfeldt-Jakob
Disease (CJD)

**Not dreaded** ──────────────────────────────────────── **Dreaded**

not catastrophic
not fatal
equitable
controlable
low risk to future generations
voluntary

Drinking alcohol
Riding a bicycle

Handguns

catastrophic
fatal
not equitable
uncontrollable
risk to future generations
involuntary

**Known risk**

observable
effect immediate
old risk
risks known to science

# ANNEX 10. HOW PEOPLE PROCESS RISK INFORMATION IN HIGH-STRESS SITUATIONS

When people are stressed, they often have difficulty hearing, understanding and remembering information. The challenges for communicators are therefore to:

- overcome the barriers created by stress;
- produce accurate messages for diverse audiences under high-stress conditions; and
- achieve maximum communication effectiveness within the constraints posed by high stress.

Solutions to these challenges include developing only a limited number of key messages (ideally three or one key message with three parts) that address underlying concerns or specific questions. In addition, keeping individual key messages brief[1] will also help, as will developing messages clearly understandable by the target audience (typically at or below their average reading grade level). Additional solutions to the problems caused by high levels of stress include:

- ordering of messages so that the two most important occupy the first and last positions (note this ordering may change depending upon the audience and the context);
- citing third parties or sources of information perceived as credible by the receiving audience;
- developing key messages and supporting information that address important risk-perception factors such as trust, benefits, control, voluntariness, dread, fairness, reversibility, catastrophic potential, effects on children, memorability, morality, origin and familiarity;
- using graphics, visual aids, analogies, quotes and narratives (including personal stories) that can increase an individual's ability to receive, understand and recall a message;
- balancing a negative key message with positive, constructive or solution-oriented key messages, typically using at least three positive, constructive or solution-oriented messages to every negative one; and
- avoiding unnecessary, indefensible or non-productive words, including "never", "always" or other absolutes.

---

[1] Ideally less than 3 seconds (or less than 9 words) for each key message, and less than 9 seconds (or 27 words) for the entire set of three key messages.

# ANNEX 11. HOW PEOPLE FORM PERCEPTIONS OF TRUST

The trustworthiness of a message is typically judged by its content and by its source – "who is telling me this, and can I trust them"? If the answer to the latter is "no" the communication is likely to fail regardless of its content.

Trust can only be built up over time. It is based on a proven record of listening, caring, competence, honesty and accountability. In general, experts no longer automatically command the levels of trust observed in the past. Reliance on scientific credentials alone to establish trust is unlikely to prove effective. Building trust is a long-term, cumulative process that needs to be started well in advance of an emergency. Trust is easily lost and once lost is difficult to regain.

Research indicates that trust is more likely to be strong where:

- organizations are clear about their values and goals;
- there is openness and transparency about decisions;
- the organization is the first to announce bad news;
- early warnings have been provided;
- decisions are clearly grounded in scientific evidence;
- public values, concerns and perceptions are taken into account in decision-making;
- people perceive that authorities share their values;
- sufficient information is provided to allow individuals to make balanced, informed judgements;
- mistakes are quickly acknowledged and acted on by authorities;
- actions are consistent with words (judgements about trust often depend more on what is done than on what is said);
- uncertainty is acknowledged;
- excessive reassurance is avoided;
- others with high credibility support your statements and positions; and
- outrage and the legitimacy of fear and emotion are acknowledged.

The most important factors involved in trust include perceived:

- listening, caring, empathy and compassion;
- honesty, openness, candidness, transparency and accountability;
- expertise, competence and wisdom;
- perseverance, dedication, commitment and responsiveness; and
- objectivity, fairness and consistency.

# SELECTED READING
## INTERNATIONAL PERSPECTIVES AND CULTURAL DIVERSITY

Astrom AN, Awadia AK, Bjorvatn K. Perceptions of susceptibility to oral health hazards: a study of women in different cultures. *Community Dentistry and Oral Epidemiology*, 1999, August, 27(4):268–274.

Ayish M. Risk communication: a cross-cultural study. *European Journal of Communication*, 1991, June, 6(2):213–222.

Calman KC, Royston GHD. Risk Language and Dialects. *British Medical Journal*, 1997, 315:939–942.

Douglas M, Wildavsky A. *Risk and Culture: An Essay on the Selection of Technological and Environmental Dangers*. University of California Press, 1983.

el Katsha S, Watts S. Schistosomiasis in two Nile delta villages: an anthropological perspective. *Tropical Medicine and International Health*, 1997, 2(9):846–854.

Finucane ML, Maybery MT. Risk perceptions in Australia. *Psychological Reports*, 1996, December, 79(3 Part 2):1331–1338.

Haider M. *Global Public Health Communication: Challenges, Perspectives and Strategies*. Jones and Bartlett Publishers, Sudbury, Massachusetts, 2005.

Hoeman SP, Ku YL, Ohl DR. Health beliefs and early detection among Chinese women. *Western Journal of Nursing Research*, 1996, 18(5):518–533.

Huerta EE, Macario E. Communicating health risk to ethnic groups: reaching Hispanics as a case study. *Journal of the National Cancer Institute Monographs*, 1999, (25):23–26.

Jianguang Z. Environmental hazards in the Chinese public's eyes. *Risk Analysis*, 1993, October, 13(5):509–513.

Johnson BB, Covello V. *The social and cultural construction of risk: Essays on risk selection and perception*. D Reidel Publishing Company, Boston, Massachusetts, 1987.

Kasperson RE, Stallen PJ, eds. *Communicating risks to the public: international perspectives*. Boston, Kluwer Academic Publishers, 1991.

Krishnatray PK, Melkote SR. Public communication campaigns in the destigmatization of leprosy: a comparative analysis of diffusion and participatory approaches. A case study in Gwalior, India. *Journal of Health Communication*, 1998, October-December, 3(4):327–344.

Lau J, Tsui H, Kim J. Monitoring community responses to the SARS epidemic in Hong Kong: from day 10 to day 62. *Journal of Epidemiology and Community Health*, 2003, 57(11):864–870.

Lipkus IM, Hollands JG. The visual communication of risk. *Journal of the National Cancer Institute Monographs*, 1999, (25):149–163.

Liu JT, Smith VK. Risk communication and attitude change: Taiwan national debate over nuclear power. *Journal of Risk and Uncertainty*, 1990, December, 3(4):331–349.

Lofstedt RE. Risk communication in the Swedish energy sector. *Energy Policy*, 1993, July, 21(7):768–772.

# HEALTH, RISK AND EMERGENCY COMMUNICATIONS

Bennett P, Calman K, eds. *Risk communication and public health*. New York (NY), Oxford University Press, 1999.

Bryant GD, Norman GR. Expressions of probability: Words and numbers. *New England Journal of Medicine*, 1980, February, 302(7):411.

Centers for Disease Control and Prevention. *Emergency Risk Communication. CDCynergy* (CD-ROM). Atlanta, 2004.

Chartier J, Gabler S. *Risk communication and government: theory and application for the Canadian Food Inspection Agency*. Canadian Food Inspection Agency Public and Regulatory Affairs Branch, 2001.

Chess C, Hance BJ, Sandman PM. *Planning dialogue with communities: a risk communication workbook*. New Brunswick, New Jersey, Rutgers University, Cook College, Environmental Media Communication Research Program. 1989.

Cohn LD et al. Adolescents' misinterpretation of health risk probability expressions. *Pediatrics*, 1995, May, 95(5):713–716.

Covello V, Allen F. *Seven cardinal rules of risk communication*. Washington, DC, United States Environmental Protection Agency, 1988.

Covello VT. Communicating information about the health risks of radioactive waste: a review of obstacles to public understanding. *Bulletin of the New York Academy of Medicine*, 1989, April-May, 65(4):467–482.

Covello, VT. Best practice in public health risk and crisis communication. *Journal of Health Communication*, 2003, 8 Supplement 1:5–8.

Covello VT, McCallum DB, Pavlova MT, eds. *Effective risk communication: the role and responsibility of government and non-government organizations*. New York, Plenum Press, 1989.

Covello VT et al. Risk communication, the West Nile virus epidemic, and bioterrorism: responding to the communication challenges posed by the intentional or unintentional release of a pathogen in an urban setting. *Journal of Urban Health*, 2001, June, 78(2):382–391.

Covello VT, Sandman PM. Risk communication: evolution and revolution. In: Wolbarst A, ed. *Solutions to an Environment in Peril*. Baltimore, Maryland, Johns Hopkins University Press, 2001, 164–178.

Cvetkovich G, Lofstedt R, eds. *Social trust and the management of risk*. London, Earthscan Publications, 2000.

de Bruin WB et al. Verbal and numerical expressions of probability: "it's a fifty-fifty chance". *Organizational Behavior and Human Decision Processes*, 2000, January, 81(1):115–131.

Department of Health and Human Services (United States). *Communicating in a crisis: Risk communication guidelines for public officials*. Washington, DC, 2002.

Fischhoff B. Risk perception and communication unplugged: twenty years of process. *Risk Analysis*, 1995, April, 15(2):137–145.

Fischhoff B, Bostrom A, Quadrel MJ. Risk perception and communication. *Annual Review of Public Health*, 1993, 14:183–203.

Fisher A, Pavlova M, Covello V, eds. *Evaluation and effective risk communication*. Washington, Interagency Task Force on Environmental Cancer and Heart and Lung Disease, 1989.

Freimuth V, Linnan HW, Potter P. Communicating the threat of emerging infections to the public. *Emerging Infectious Diseases*, 2000, July-August, 6(4):337–347. Erratum in: *Emerging Infectious Diseases*, 2001, January-February, 7(1):167.

Grabenstein JD, Wilson JP. Are vaccines safe? Risk communication applied to vaccines. *Hospital Pharmacy*, 1999, 34:713–714; 717–718; 721–723; 727–729.

Health and Safety Executive (UK). *Risk communication: a guide to regulatory practice*. Inter-Departmental Group on Risk Assessment, Health and Safety Executive, London, 1998.

Hobbs J et al. Communicating health information to an alarmed public facing a threat such as a bioterrorist attack. *Journal of Health Communication*, 2004, January-February, 9(1):67–75.

Jungermann H, Wiedemann PM. Risk communication – introduction. *European Review of Applied Psychology*, 1995, 45(1):3–5.

Kahnemann D, Tversky A. Prospect theory: An analysis of decision under risk. *Econometrica*, 1979, 47(2):263–291.

Krimsky S, Golding D, eds. *Societal Theories of Risk*. Praeger, New York, 1992.

Krimsky S, Plough A. *Environmental Hazards: Communicating Risks as a Social Process*. Dover, MA, Auburn House, 1988.

Lakey J. Informing the public about radiation – the messenger and the message: 1997. *Health Physics*, 1998, October, 75(4):367–374.

Leiss W. Three phases in the evolution of risk communication practice. *The Annals of the American Academy of Political and Social Science*, 1996, May, 545:85–94.

Lum MR, Tinker TL. *A primer on health risk communication principles and practices*. Washington, DC, Agency for Toxic Substances and Disease Registry (United States), United States Government Printing Office, Washington, DC, no: HE 20.502:97024783, 1994.

Lundgren R, McMakin A. *Risk communication: a handbook for communicating environmental, safety, and health risks*. 3rd ed. Columbus, Ohio, Batelle Press, 2004.

Maibach E, Holtgrave DR. Advances in public health communication. *Annual Review of Public Health*, 1995, 16:219–238.

McNeil BJ et al. On the elicitation of preferences for alternative therapies. *New England Journal of Medicine*, 1982, May, 306(21):1259–1262.

Morgan GM et al. *Risk communication: a mental models approach*. Cambridge, Cambridge University Press, 2001.

Morgan G et al. Communicating risk to the public. *Environmental Science and Technology*, 1992, 26(11):2048–2056.

National Health Service (UK), Department of Health. *Communicating about risks to public health: pointers to good practice*. London, United Kingdom Department of Health, 1997.

National Research Council (US). *Improving risk communication*. Committee on Risk Perception and Risk Communication. Washington, DC, National Academy Press, 1989.

## SELECTED READING

Nicholson PJ. Communicating health risk. *Occupational Medicine*, 1999, May, 49(4):253–256.

Noll AM, ed. *Crisis communications: Lessons from September 11*. Lanham, Maryland, Rowman & Littlefield Publishers, 2004.

Pan American Health Organization. *Communicating with the public in times of disaster: guidelines for disaster managers on preparing and disseminating effective health messages*. Pan American Health Organization, Caribbean Office, Barbados, 1994.

Peters RG, Covello VT, McCallum DB. The determinants of trust and credibility in environmental risk communication: An empirical study. *Risk Analysis*, 1997, 17(1):43–54.

Peterson L, Specht E, Wight E. *The Technical Basis for the [United States] NRC's Guidelines for External Risk Communication*. Washington, United States Nuclear Regulatory Commission (NUREG/CR-6840), 2004.

Pollard, WE. Public perceptions of information sources concerning bioterrorism before and after anthrax attacks: An analysis of national survey data. *Journal of Health Communication*, 2003, 8 Supplement 1:93–103

Powell D, Leiss W. *Mad Cows and Mother's Milk: The Perils of Poor Risk Communication*. Montreal, Canada, McGill-Queen's University Press, 1997.

Quarantelli EL. The sociology of panic. In: Smelser N, Baltes PB, eds. *International encyclopedia of the social and behavioral sciences*. New York, Pergamon, 2001, 20–30.

Ratzan SC. Strategic health communication and social marketing on risk issues. Journal of Health Communication, 1999, January-March, 4(1):1–6.

Renn O, Levine D. Credibility and trust in risk communication. In: Kasperson RE, Stallen PJM, eds. *Communicating Risks to the Public: International Perspectives*. Dordrecht, Kluwer Academic Publishers, 1991, 175–219.

Renn O et al. The social amplification of risk: Theoretical foundations and empirical applications. *Journal of Social Science Issues*, 1992, 48:137–160.

Ropeik D, Gray G. *Risk: A Practical Guide for Deciding What's Really Safe and What's Really Dangerous in the World around You*. Boston, Massachusetts, Houghton Mifflin, 2002.

Rothman AJ, Kiviniemi MT. Treating people with information: an analysis and review of approaches to communicating health risk information. *Journal of the National Cancer Institute Monographs*, 1999, 25:44–51.

Rowe WD et al. *Evaluation Methods for Environmental Standards*. Boca Raton, Florida, CRC Press, 1984.

Royal Society. *Risk: Analysis, Perception, Management*. London, 1992.

Sandman PM. Hazard versus outrage in the public perception of risk. In: Covello VT, McCallum DB, Pavlova MT, eds. *Effective Risk communication: The Role and Responsibility of Government and Nongovernment Organizations*. New York, NY, Plenum Press, 1989, 45–49.

Sandman PM, Lanard J. *Risk communication recommendations for infectious disease outbreaks*. Invited Paper. World Health Organization SARS Scientific Research Advisory Committee meeting, 20–21 October 2003, Geneva.

Schulte PA, Singal M. Interpretation and communication of the results of medical field investigations. *Journal of Occupational Medicine*, 1989, July 31(7):589–594.

Slovic P. Informing and educating the public about risk. *Risk Analysis*, 1986, December, 6(4):403–415.

Slovic P. Perception of risk. *Science*, 1987, 236:280–285.

Slovic P, Krauss N, Covello V. What should we know about making risk comparisons?. *Risk Analysis*, 1990, 10:389–392.

Sublet VH, Covello VT, Tinker TL, eds. *Scientific uncertainty and its influence on the public communication process*. Boston, Kluwer Academic Publishers, 1996.

Swedish Emergency Management Agency. *Crisis communication handbook*. Stockholm, 2003.

Tinker T, Silberberg P. *US Agency for Toxic Substances and Disease Registry Evaluation primer on health risk communication programs*. US Department of Health and Human Services, 1997.

Tversky A, Kahneman D. Judgement under uncertainty: Heuristics and biases. *Science*, 1974, 185:1124–1131.

Williams D, Olaniran BA. Expanding the crisis planning function: introducing elements of risk communication to crisis communication planning. *Public Relations Review*, 1998, 24(3):401–412.

Witte K, Allen M. A meta-analysis of fear appeals: implications for effective public health campaigns. *Health Education and Behavior*, 2000, 27:591–615.

Witte K. Generating effective risk messages: How scary should your risk communication be? *Communication Yearbook*, 1994, 18:229–254.

**SELECTED READING**

# MEDIA COMMUNICATION AND PUBLIC HEALTH

Bellicha T, McGrath J. Mass media approaches to reducing cardiovascular disease risk. *Public Health Reports*, 1990, May-June, 105:245–252.

Boffey PM, Rodgers JE, Schneider SH. Interpreting uncertainty: a panel discussion. In: Friedman SM, Dunwoody S, Rogers CL, eds. *Communicating uncertainty: media coverage of new and controversial science*. Mahwah, New Jersey, Lawrence Erlbaum Associates, Inc, 1999, 81–91.

Brody JE. Communicating cancer risk in print journalism. *Journal of the National Cancer Institute Monographs*, 1999, 25:170–172.

Chipman H et al. Audience responses to a risk communication message in four media formats. *Journal of Nutrition Education*, 1996, May-June, 28(3):133–139.

Coleman CL. The influence of mass media and interpersonal communication on societal and personal risk judgments. *Communication Research*, 1993, August, 20(4):611–618.

Dearing JW, Rogers EM. AIDS and the media agenda. In: Edgar T, Fitzpatrick MA, eds. *AIDS: a communication perspective*. Hillsdale, New Jersey, Lawrence Erlbaum Associates, Inc, 1992, 173–194.

Dooley KJ, Corman SR. The dynamics of electronic media coverage. In: Greenberg BS, ed. *Communication and terrorism: Public and media responses to 9/11*. Cresskill, New Jersey, Hampton Press, 2002, 121–135.

Dornan C. Some problems in conceptualizing the issue of science and the media. *Critical Studies in Mass Communication*, 1990, March, 7(1):48–71.

Dunwoody S, Ryan M. Public information persons as mediators between scientists and journalists. *Journalism Quarterly*, 1983, 60:647–656.

Dunwoody S, Scott B. Scientists as mass media sources. *Journalism Quarterly*, 1982, 59:52–59.

Dunwoody S. Scientists, journalists, and the meaning of uncertainty. In: Friedman SM, Dunwoody S, Rogers CL, eds. *Communicating uncertainty: media coverage of new and controversial science*. Mahwah, New Jersey, Lawrence Erlbaum Associates, Inc, 1999, 59–79.

Einsiedel E, Thorne B. Public responses to uncertainty. In: Friedman SM, Dunwoody S, Rogers CL, eds. *Communicating uncertainty: media coverage of new and controversial science*. Mahwah, New Jersey, Lawrence Erlbaum Associates, Inc, 1999, 43–57.

Eldridge J, Reilly J. Risk and relativity: BSE and the British media. In: Pidgeon N, Kasperson RE, Slovic P, eds. *The social amplification of risk*. Cambridge, Cambridge University Press, 2003, 138–155.

Finer D, Tomson G, Bjorkman NM. Ally, advocate, analyst, agenda-setter? Positions and perceptions of Swedish medical journalists. *Patient Education and Counseling*, 1997, January, 30(1):71–81.

Freudenburg WR et al. Media coverage of hazard events: analyzing the assumptions. *Risk Analysis*, 1996, February, 16(1):31–42.

Friedman SM, Dunwoody S, Rogers CL, eds. *Communicating uncertainty: media coverage of new and controversial science*. Mahwah, New Jersey, Lawrence Erlbaum Associates, Inc, 1999.

Gelb BD, Boutwell WB, Cummings S. Using mass media communication for health promotion: results from a cancer center effort. *Hospital and Health Services Administration*, 1994, Fall, 39(3):283–293.

Gunter B, Kinderlerer J, Beyleveld D. The media and public understanding of biotechnology. *Science Communication*, 1999, June, 20(4):373–394.

Houn F et al. The association between alcohol and breast cancer: popular press coverage of research. *American Journal of Public Health*, 1995, August, 85(8, Part 1):1082–1086.

Kittler A et al. The Internet as a vehicle to communicate health information during a public health emergency: A survey analysis involving the anthrax scare of 2001. *Journal of Medical Internet Research*, 2004, 6(1):75–81

Lanouette W. Reporting on risk: Who decides what's news? *Risk*, 1994, Summer, 5:223–232.

Levine J. Risky business – communicating scientific findings to the public. *Journal of the National Cancer Institute Monographs*, 1999, (25):163–166.

Mazur A. Technical risk in the mass media. *Risk*, 1994, Summer, 5:189

Mebane F, Temin S, Parvanta CF. Communicating anthrax in 2001: A comparison of CDC information and print media accounts. *Journal of Health Communication*, 2003, 8:50–82.

Mullin S. The anthrax attacks in New York City: The "Giuliani press conference model" and other communication strategies that helped. *Journal of Health Communication*, 2003, 8:15–16.

National Safety Council (US), Environmental Health Center. *Chemicals, the press & the public: a journalists' guide to reporting on chemicals in the community*. 2nd edition. Washington, DC, Environmental Health Center, National Safety Council, 2000.

Peters HP. The interaction of journalists and scientific experts: cooperation and conflict between two professional cultures. *Media, Culture, & Society*, 1995, January, 17(1):31–48.

Peters HP. Mass media as an information channel and public arena. *Risk*, 1994, Summer, 5:241.

Rezza G, Marino R, Farchi F. SARS: The epidemic in the press. *Emerging Infectious Diseases*, 2004, 10:381–382.

Robinson SJ, Newstetter WC. Uncertain science and certain deadlines: CDC responses to the media during the anthrax attacks of 2001. *Journal of Health Communication*, 2003, 8:17–34.

Roche JP, Muskavitch MAT. Limited precision in print media communication of West Nile virus risks. *Science Communication*, 2003, 24:353–365.

Rogers CL. The importance of understanding audiences. In: Friedman SM, Dunwoody S, Rogers CL, eds. *Communicating uncertainty: media coverage of new and controversial science*. Mahwah, New Jersey, Lawrence Erlbaum Associates, Inc,1999, 179–200.

Rogers EM. Diffusion of news of the September 11 terrorist attacks. In: Noll AM, ed. *Crisis communications: Lessons from September 11*. Lanham, Maryland, Rowman & Littlefield, 2003, 7–30.

Rowan KE. Explaining illness through the mass media: the problem-solving perspective. In: Whaley BB et al., eds. *Explaining illness: research, theory, and strategies*. Mahwah, New Jersey, Lawrence Erlbaum Associates, Inc, 2000, 69–100.

Rowe G, Frewer L, Sjoberg L. Newspaper reporting of hazards in the UK and Sweden. *Public Understanding of Science*, 2000, January 9(1):59–78.

Russell C. Living can be hazardous to your health: how the news media cover cancer risks.

*Journal of the National Cancer Institute Monographs*, 1999, (25):167–70.

Sandman PM. Mass media and environmental risk: seven principles. *Risk*, 1994, 5:251.

Scanlon E, Whitelegg E, Yates S, eds. *Communicating science. Vol. 1: Contexts and channels.* London, Routledge, 1999.

Singer E, Endreny PM. *Reporting on risk: how the mass media portray accidents, diseases, disasters and other hazards.* New York, New York: Russell Sage Foundation. 1993.

Stocking SH. How journalists deal with scientific uncertainty. In: Friedman SM, Dunwoody S, Rogers CL, eds. *Communicating uncertainty: media coverage of new and controversial science.* Mahwah, NJ, Lawrence Erlbaum Associates, Inc, 1999, 23–41.

Tassew A. *Reporting a pandemic: a comparative study of AIDS news coverage in African and European prestige dailies.* Dissertation. Goteborg, Goteborgs Universitet, Institutionen for Journalistik och Masskommunikation, 1995.

Willis WJ, Okunade AA. *Reporting on risks: the practice and ethics of health and safety communication.* Westport, Connecticut, Praeger, 1997.

World Health Organization. *Partnership building with the media – a workshop for national immunization managers and national regulatory authorities.* Geneva, 1999 (WHO/CDS/2005.28).